Reviewers

Aris Andrews, RN, MS
Creighton University School of Nursing, Hastings Campus
Hastings, Nevada

Susan J. Garbutt, DNP, RN, CIC
Galen School of Nursing
St. Petersburg, Florida

NOTES

INFECTION CONTROL AND PREVENTION BASICS

Importance of Infection Control and Prevention (IC)

Emergence of New Pathogens

The emergence of new pathogens (e.g., severe acute respiratory syndrome-associated coronavirus [SARS-CoV], avian influenza), threat of evolving known pathogens (e.g., *Clostridium difficile* [*C. difficile*] noroviruses), and increasing concerns for the threat of bioweapons attacks (e.g., smallpox and anthrax) have established a great need to reemphasize infection control and prevention.[1]

Healthcare-Associated Infections

A continued increase in the incidence of healthcare-associated infections (HAIs)—especially those caused by multidrug-resistant organisms (MDROs)—and the expanded body of knowledge related to preventing transmission of MDROs have created a need for more specific recommendations for surveillance and prevention of these pathogens.[1]

HAIs lead to lawsuits and increase morbidity, mortality, medical expenses, and economic cost.[5] Hospital administrators and the general public are more aware than ever before of the need for infection control and prevention. Healthcare-associated infections, however, are preventable.

Patient Safety

Patient safety has been given increased scrutiny by the Joint Commission, which considers HAIs to be a patient-safety issue. The Joint Commission's 2009 National Patient Safety Goal 7 (NPSG 7)[2] addresses reducing the risk of healthcare-associated infections in three important ways:

- Meeting hand hygiene guidelines (NPSG 07.01.01)

- Managing as sentinel events all identified cases of unanticipated death or major permanent loss of function related to healthcare-associated infection (NPSG 07.02.01)

- Implementing evidence-based practices to prevent healthcare-associated infection due to multidrug-resistant organisms in acute care hospitals (NPSG 07.03.01)

New Rules: Pay for Performance

Hospitals will no longer be paid for eight conditions presented by the Centers for Medicare and Medicaid Services (CMS). Three of the eight conditions are HAIs: catheter-associated urinary tract infection, vascular catheter-associated infection, and surgical site infection/mediastinitis after coronary artery bypass graft.[3]

In October 2008, CMS added three additional hospital-acquired conditions to the new final rule, for a total of eleven conditions. One of the three additional conditions is surgical site infection following bariatric surgery for obesity and certain orthopedic surgeries including repair, replacement, or fusion of joints of shoulder, elbow, and spine.

Consumers Union is encouraging legislatures to enact state laws requiring public disclosure of hospital infection rates.[4]

Continuing Education for Nurses

Nurses in all specialties are on the frontline in the never-ending war against infectious diseases and pathogens. Nurses must know what precautions to take while caring for patients with infections. Healthcare providers must be aware of the principles of infection control and prevention to protect themselves from occupational exposure and to protect their patients from being exposed to pathogens. Nurses who decide placement of newly admitted patients must know how to assign patients with infections.

Effective patient safety and infection control and prevention programs require that healthcare providers be familiar with recent Centers for Disease Control and Prevention (CDC) recommendations, understand the evidence behind those recommendations, and consistently adhere to the recommendations.

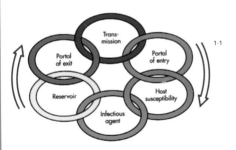

1-1

Chain of Infection

Principles of Infection

Infection Process

Chain of Infection

The Chain of Infection is a model used to describe the infection process. There are six links in this chain, with the first and last linked to form a circle named the *Chain of Infection*.[6,7] Each link in this chain is a component of the infectious disease process. For an infection to occur, all links in the chain must be present. Break any link, and infection cannot occur. Therefore understanding each of these links can help healthcare workers (HCWs) protect both patients and themselves. The six links in the Chain of Infection are: infectious agent, reservoir, portal of exit, mode of transmission, portal of entry, and host susceptibility—bringing us full circle.

Components of Chain of Infection and Explanations[6,5]

Components of Chain of Infection	Explanations	Example: Pulmonary tuberculosis
Infectious agent	Biological agents: bacteria, viruses, fungi, protozoa, prions	Mycobacterium tuberculosis complex
Reservoir	Place where an infectious agent can survive but may or may not reproduce (e.g., human, animal, environment)	Primarily human; in some areas, infected animals, e.g., cattle, badgers, and other mammals
Portal of exit	Path by which the infectious agent leaves the reservoir (e.g., respiratory tract, gastrointestinal tract, genitourinary tract, skin/mucous membrane, blood, transplacental)	Tubercle bacilli in airborne droplet nuclei (tiny and very light, about 1-5 μm in size) produced by patients with pulmonary or respiratory tract tuberculosis during expiratory efforts, e.g., coughing, singing, shouting, or sneezing
Mode of transmission	How the infectious agent reaches a susceptible host (e.g., contact, droplet, airborne transmission)	Exposure to tubercle bacilli in airborne droplet nuclei

Components of Chain of Infection and Explanations (cont'd)

Portal of entry	Path by which the infectious agent enters the reservoir (e.g., respiratory tract, gastrointestinal tract, genitourinary tract, skin/mucous membrane, blood, transplacental)	Tubercle bacilli in airborne droplet nuclei inhaled into pulmonary alveolae

Host susceptibility	Host's characteristics influencing susceptibility to infectious agents (e.g., age, medical condition, trauma, occupation)	• The risk of infection is directly related to the degree of exposure and does not appear related to genetics or race.
		  • Children
		  • Elderly
		  • HIV infected patients
		  • Immunosuppressed patients
		  • Patients with debilitating disorder, e.g., chronic renal failure, cancer, diabetes.
		  • Underweight or undernourished people

Infectious Agents[8,9]

1. Bacteria

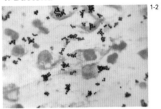

Clusters of gram-positive cocci in a patient with *Staphylococcus aureus* pneumonia

Characteristics

- A unicellular microorganism with no nucleus

- Classification: prokaryotes

- Four major shapes:
    1. coccus (plural: cocci): spherical
    2. bacillus (plural: bacilli): rods; short bacilli are called coccobacilli
    3. spiral forms: common-shaped, S-shaped, spiral-shaped, vibrio
    4. pleomorphic: lacking a shape

The degree of virulence depends on cell structures such as flagella, pili, capsules, endospores, and biofilms (extracellular polysaccharide network).

Examples

- *Staphylococcus aureus*—causes surgical site infection, cellulitis, sepsis, pneumonia. When S. aureus develops resistance to oxacillin/methicillin, it is called MRSA (methicillin-resistant Staphylococcus aureus)

- *Clostridium difficile*—causes diarrhea, colitis, colon perforation

2. Viruses

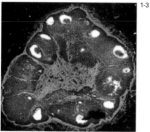
1-3

Lymph node infected with *HIV (human immunodeficiency virus)*, seen in this specially stained micrograph as white areas.

Characteristics

- Viruses are the simplest and smallest known forms of life.

- Unlike most bacteria, which can grow on nonliving surfaces, viruses require a living host to multiply.

- Unlike bacteria, viruses are unable to replicate on their own. The virus must invade a living cell (host) and use the cell's internal machinery to reproduce itself. The host cell is destroyed or damaged by this process. Viruses carry only genetic information, either DNA or RNA, never both.

Examples

- Human immunodeficiency virus (HIV)—causes acquired immune deficiency syndrome (AIDS)

- Hepatitis B and hepatitis C viruses—cause hepatitis B and hepatitis C, liver cirrhosis, liver failure, even hepatocellular carcinoma (HCC)

3. Fungi

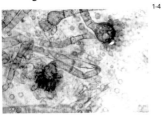

Fruiting head of *Aspergillus fumigatus* on a lung biopsy.

Characteristics

- Fungi are eukaryotic organisms deriving nutrients from organic materials.

- Fungi are typically classified as either yeasts or molds.

- Most fungal pathogens are acquired through contact with airborne spores or decaying organic matter in the environment.

  Examples

- *Candida* species (yeasts)—cause mucositis, vaginitis, dermatitis, systemic or disseminated candidiasis

- *Cryptococcus neoformans* (yeasts)— cause meningitis, pneumonia in immunocompromised hosts

- *Aspergillus* species (mold)—cause necrotizing pneumonia

4. Parasites

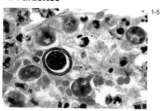
1-5

This photomicrograph depicted a magnified view of brain tissue within which was a centrally located *Acanthamoeba sp.* cyst. *Acanthamoeba spp.* are opportunistic free-living amebae, capable of causing granulomatous amebic encephalitis (GAE) in individuals with compromised immune systems.

Characteristics

- Parasites may be single-celled microscopic protozoa or complex worms several feet long.

- Protozoa are unicellular, free-living eukaryotic organisms.

Protozoa exist in two forms: the pleomorphic trophozoite stage and the cysts stage (most responsible for transmission).

Examples

- Giardia lamblia—causes watery diarrhea, intestinal malabsorption

- Amoeba—causes fulminant colitis, dysentery, liver abscess

Fighting Infections

Infection Control and Prevention Program

Preventing infection requires a team effort by administrators, HCWs, non-HCWs, patients, and visitors. In most healthcare settings, there is a department of Infection control and prevention to monitor HAI rate, standardize infection control practice, and coordinate with various departments.

- The core personnel of the IC program are the infection control practitioner (ICP) and chair of the IC committee (usually an infectious disease physician with epidemiology training). The IC committee is a multidisciplinary team.

- The principal functions of an infection control and prevention program include but are not limited to:
  1. Managing and obtaining critical surveillance data for hospital-associated infections
  2. Developing and recommending infection control–related policies and procedures
  3. Intervening directly to prevent infections
  4. Investigating outbreaks
  5. Managing occupational exposures
  6. Communicating with local Department of Public Health about reportable communicable diseases (varies by state), any novel organisms, and outbreaks
  7. Educating and training HCWs, non-HCWs, volunteers, patients, and families
  8. Providing infection control consultation

- Hospital leadership can positively impact HCW adherence to recommended infection control practices. Several administrative factors may shape infection control and prevention in healthcare settings: institutional culture, working environment, individual HCW behavior, and safety culture within the organization.

- Education and training of HCWs and non-HCWs are necessary to ensure that policies and procedures for standard and transmission-based precautions are understood and implemented. Understanding the scientific rationale for the precautions will help HCWs correctly comply with policies and procedures.

- Professionals in the safety, maintenance, and employee health departments play a vital role in infection control and prevention. Safety and maintenance departments should work together to provide a safe working environment and to ensure employee safety. Employee health departments should review immunization prior to employment, manage occupational exposure, track sharp injuries, and offer vaccines and PPD tests.

- The Occupational Safety and Health Administration (OSHA) mandates a Respiratory Protection Program. Components of such a program include medical clearance for the wearing of respirators, use of appropriate respirators (including fit-tested NIOSH-certified N95 and higher particulate filtering respirators), respirator use education, and periodic respiratory protection program re-evaluation. All HCWs in settings containing airborne infection isolation rooms (AIIRs) require fit-testing. Optimal fit-testing frequency has not been determined by the CDC; most healthcare settings repeat fit-testing for HCWs on an annual basis. Retesting may be needed if facial features change, if HCWs have a medical condition affecting respiratory function, or if the size or model of the initially assigned respirator is changed. Fit-testing does not apply to patients and visitors.[1]

- ICPs should identify cases with reportable illness quickly. ICPs must then collect and report data to the local departments of public health. After gathering data from each state, the CDC may publish the study as below.

[1-5]

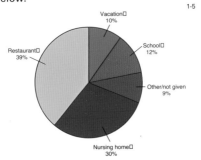

Settings for 348 outbreaks of Norwalk-like viruses reported to CDC, 1996-2000.

- Patients, visitors and family members should be encouraged to partner with HCWs to help prevent transmission of infections in healthcare settings. To help enlist them in this effort, they should be given the knowledge needed to play their part. Education should be provided on complying with standard and transmission-based precautions, hand hygiene, respiratory hygiene/cough etiquette (covering the nose/mouth with tissue when sneezing/coughing, promptly disposing of used tissue, using surgical masks when tolerated and appropriate on the coughing person), and vaccination (particularly during influenza season). These and other routine infection prevention strategies may be incorporated into patient education materials provided upon admission to the healthcare facility.

- Visitor Management[1]:
  1. All visitors should be instructed and encouraged to comply with hand hygiene and respiratory hygiene/cough etiquette.

  2. Visitor screening is essential, particularly during community outbreaks of infectious diseases. Healthcare facilities should develop an effective visitor screening program to limit hospital visitation by the people with signs or symptoms of a communicable infection.

  3. Sibling visits are encouraged in pediatric settings. However, child visitors should visit their own siblings only. Screening of child visitors before they enter the patient rooms is necessary to prevent the introduction of childhood illnesses and common respiratory infections to the patients.

  4. In some healthcare settings, visitors are required to wear proper personal protective equipment (PPE) (e.g., gowns, gloves, or masks) before entering an isolation room. Some facilities do not address the use of PPE for visitors.

  5. Visitors should be educated on the necessity of using of PPE and encour-

aged to comply with isolation precautions, especially visitors participating in patient care (e.g. bathing, feeding) or having close patient contact (e.g., holding). Patient population and the level of interaction should determine the degree to which visitors should use PPE. In this book, the highest level of isolation precautions compliance for visitors will be outlined.

Figure References

1-1. Perry AG. Clinical Nursing Skills & Techniques. 6th ed. St Louis: Mosby; 2005.

1-2. Andreoli TE et al. Andreoli and Carpenter's Cecil Essentials of Medicine. 7th ed. Philadelphia: Saunders; 2007.

1-3. Thibodeau GA. Anatomy & Physiology. 6th ed. St Louis: Mosby; 2006.

1-4. Andreoli TE et al. Andreoli and Carpenter's Cecil Essentials of Medicine. 7th ed. Philadelphia: Saunders; 2007.

1-5. Courtesy of Centers for Disease Control and Prevention.

1-6. Data from Centers for Disease Control and Prevention. Norwalk-like viruses: public health consequences and outbreak management. MMWR, Morb Mortal Wkly Rep. 2001;50(RR-9):18. Maurer FA. Community/Public Health Nursing Practice: Health for Families and Populations. 3rd ed. Philadelphia: Saunders; 2004.

LAB TESTS TO SCREEN FOR INFECTION

Tests and Studies for Infection Process with Normal Values, *18*

Tests and Studies for Infection Process with Normal Values[10,11]

WBC Scan

Purpose

Used to identify and locate infection or inflammations. The WBCs are localized to the area of infection and increase radionuclear uptake.

Normal Adult Values

No accumulation of WBCs.

Indications

Abnormal results usually suggest an active inflammation or infection, such as an intraabdominal abscess, osteomyelitis, or sinus infection.

Antigen Detection

Purpose

Test for the presence of infectious antigens.

Normal Adult Values

Negative

Indications

This test is helpful in early diagnosis when culture results are not yet positive. Antigen testing can identify adenovirus, Neisseria meningitidis, immunodeficiency virus, and hepatitis virus.

C-Reactive Protein (CRP)

Purpose

Used to diagnose current inflammatory process.

Normal Adult Values

Negative

Indications

The liver can produce CRP, an abnormal serum glycoprotein, during acute infection. When inflammation subsides, CRP disappears.

Complete Blood Count (CBC)

Purpose

Used to screen for general health and track the progress of disease.

WBC count is useful in diagnosing and monitoring infection.

Normal Adult Values

WBC count varies, depending on age of patient. Range is typically 5000 to 10,000 per mm^3.

Indications

Increased WBC count (>10,000) is a sign of infection, inflammation, or leukemic neoplasia. Decreased WBC count (<4000) may occur in cases of overwhelming infections such as viral hepatitis and AIDS.

Body Fluid Analysis

Purpose

Used to test for infection in a body fluid (e.g., pleural fluid, peritoneal fluid).

Normal Adult Values

Varies with type of body fluid. Analysis includes Gram stain, cell counts, total protein, and specific gravity.

Indications

Presence of WBCs in large numbers is a sign of infection and acute inflammation.

Cerebrospinal Fluid (CSF) Analysis

Purpose

Used to diagnose meningitis.

Normal Adult Values

Four components—color/clarity, protein, glucose, and WBC count—are used to diagnose infection.

Indications

Indication of bacterial meningitis:

- CSF color/clarity: cloudy

- Protein: high

- Glucose: low

- WBCs: high

Urinalysis

Purpose

Used to assess general health and health of the urinary tract.

Normal Adult Values

Urinalysis includes several components: color/clarity, glucose, protein, ketones, and nitrite. The urine is also tested microscopically for RBCs, WBCs, casts, crystals, bacteria, pus cells, and yeast. A WBC count greater than 10 in the urine may indicate infection. The nitrite test is used to screen for the presence of bacteria in urine. Many bacteria produce an enzyme that can reduce urinary nitrates to nitrites.

Indications

Positive leukocyte esterase test indicates WBCs in the urine. Subsequent microscopic examination showing 10 or more WBCs may be a sign of infection.

Nitrites present in the urine may indicate the presence of bacteria. Subsequent microscopic examination showing the presence of bacteria may indicate infection or colonization of the urinary tract.

Urine Culture and Sensitivity (C&S)*

Purpose

Used to identify pathogens in the urinary tract and to guide antimicrobial therapy.

Normal Adult Values

Negative

Indications

- Positive urine culture (≥100,000 CFU/mL) indicates UTI.

- Positive urine culture (≤100,000 CFU/mL) with no signs/symptoms indicates asymptomatic colonization.

Sputum Culture and Sensitivity (C&S)*

Purpose

Used to identify pathogens in the respiratory tract and to guide antimicrobial therapy.

Normal Adult Values

Growth of normal respiratory flora only.

Indications

- Positive sputum culture indicates either infection or colonization of the respiratory tract.

- Patients infected with pathogens will have a positive sputum culture and clinical signs/symptoms of pulmonary infection and an abnormal chest x-ray.

- Patients colonized with pathogens will have a positive sputum culture but be without clinical signs/symptoms of pulmonary infection.

Blood Culture and Sensitivity (C&S)*

Purpose

Used to identify bacterial or fungi in the bloodstream and to guide antimicrobial therapy.

Normal Adult Values

Negative. No growth of microorganisms because bloodstream should be sterile.

Indications

- Positive blood culture indicates sepsis or bacteremia

Stool Culture and Sensitivity (C&S)*

Purpose

Used to identify pathogens in the bowel.

Normal Adult Values

Growth of normal intestinal flora.

Indications

Normally, stool contains bacteria and fungi (e.g., *Escherichia coli*). The normal stool flora can become pathogenic if overgrowth of the bacteria occurs due to antibiotics or immuno-suppression. However, many organisms in the bowel act as pathogens, including *Campylobacter*, *Salmonella*, *Clostridium difficile*, and *Shigella*.

Fecal Leukocytes

Purpose

Used to determine whether pathogen responsible for diarrhea is invasive or noninvasive to the mucosa of the colon.

Normal Adult Values

No presence of leukocytes in stool.

Indications

The pathogen causing diarrhea is breaking the mucosal barrier of the colon.

All cultures should be collected prior to giving antibiotics.

Differential Count

White blood cell differential count (percentage of each type of WBC)

Neutrophils

- 55% to 70%

- Increases during acute suppurative infections

- Decreases during overwhelming bacterial infections in older adults

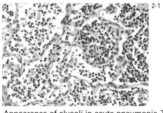

2-1

Appearance of alveoli in acute pneumonia. The alveolar walls are thickened and the spaces filled with a fibrin exudate and neutrophils (pus)—a classic finding in acute pneumonia.

Lymphocytes

- 20% to 40%

- Increases during chronic bacterial and viral infections

- Decreases during sepsis

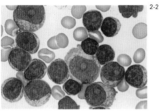

2-2

Chronic lymphocytic leukemia (CLL). Peripheral blood smear showing large numbers of diseased B lymphocytes.

Monocytes

- 2% to 8 %

- Increases during protozoal, rickettsial, and tuberculosis infections

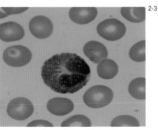

2-3

Monocytes in peripheral blood.

Eosinophils

- 1% to 4%
- Increases during parasitic infections

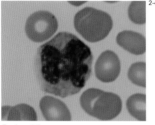

2-4

Eosinophils.

Figure References

2-1. Thibodeau GA. Anatomy & Physiology. 6th ed. St Louis: Mosby; 2006.

2-2. Thibodeau GA. Anatomy & Physiology. 6th ed. St Louis: Mosby; 2006.

2-3. Courtesy of Robert J. Homer, MD, PhD. Andreoli TE. Andreoli and Carpenter's Cecil Essentials of Medicine. 7th ed. Philadelphia: Saunders; 2007.

2-4. Andreoli TE et al. Andreoli and Carpenter's Cecil Essentials of Medicine. 7th ed. Philadelphia: Saunders; 2007.

NOTES

HAND HYGIENE

Introduction to Hand Hygiene

The goal of this section is to provide information to successfully implement the CDC 2002 "Guidelines for Hand Hygiene in Health-Care Settings" and the WHO "Guidelines on Hand Hygiene in Health Care" to meet the Joint Commission's National Patient Safety Goal (NPSG) 07.01.01.

NPSG 07.01.01 will be surveyed through interviews with caregiver staff and direct observation. Staff should understand and consistently comply with hand hygiene expectations. If surveyors observe three or more instances of noncompliance during tracer activities, a Requirement for Improvement (RFI) should result.[14]

Rationale for NPSG 07.01.01 is that complying with WHO and CDC hand hygiene guidelines will reduce the transmission of infectious agents by staff to patients, thereby decreasing the incidence of healthcare-associated infections.[2,14]

Each of the CDC recommendations is categorized on the basis of the strength of evidence supporting the recommendation. All "Category I" recommendations (including Categories IA, IB, and IC) must be implemented. Category II recommendations should be considered for implementation but are not required for accreditation purposes.[12,14,15]

CDC Recommendation Categories

Category	Meaning
IA	Strongly supported by well-designed epidemiological, clinical, or experimental studies
IB	Supported by a strong theoretical rationale and by epidemiological, clinical, or experimental studies
IC	Required for implementation, as mandated by federal or state regulation or standard
II	Suggested for implementation and supported by suggestive clinical or epidemiological studies or a theoretical rationale
None	Unresolved issue. Practices for which insufficient evidence or no consensus regarding efficacy exist

CDC Guidelines for Hand Hygiene

When to Perform Hand Hygiene[12,13]

- Decontaminate hands before direct contact with patients (IB).

- Decontaminate hands before putting on sterile gloves when inserting a central intravascular catheter (IB).

- Decontaminate hands before inserting peripheral vascular catheters, indwelling urinary catheters, or other invasive devices not requiring a surgical procedure (IB).

- Decontaminate hands following contact with a patient's intact skin (e.g., when taking pulse or blood pressure or when lifting a patient) (IB).

- Decontaminate hands following contact with wound dressings, mucous membranes, body fluids or excretions, and non-intact skin, even if hands are not visibly soiled (IA).

- Decontaminate hands after removing gloves, since wearing gloves does not replace the need for hand hygiene (IB).

- Wash hands with water and an antimicrobial or non-antimicrobial soap after using a restroom and before eating (IB).

Indications for Use[12,13,14]	
Indicator	**Action**
Hands are visibly dirty or visibly contaminated with proteinaceous material or with blood or other body fluids	Wash hands with water and an antimicrobial or a non-antimicrobial soap (IA)
Routine decontamination of hands that are not visibly soiled	Use alcohol-based hand rub (IA) **or** Wash hands with an antimicrobial or a non-antimicrobial soap and water (IB)

Hand Hygiene Methods

Tip1: After contact with spores (e.g. *Clostridium difficile* or *Bacillus anthracis*), wash hands with soap and water instead of using alcohol-based hand rub since alcohol has poor activity against spores.[15]

Tip 2: *C. difficile* and *Bacillus anthracis* are types of spore-forming bacteria. The physical action of washing and rinsing hands is recommended.[1]

Tip 3: Avoid using hot water. Repeated use may increase the risk of dermatitis (IB).[12]

Soap and Water

Step 1: Wet hands

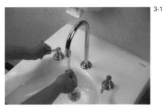

3-1

Step 2: Lather hands for 15 seconds

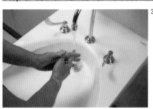

3-2

Step 3: Rinse hands with fingertips down

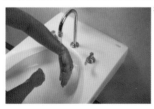

3-3

Step 4: Dry hands with clean paper towel, and use paper towel to turn off faucet

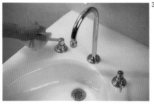

3-4

Alcohol-Based Hand Rub (IB)[12,13]

Step 1	Apply the manufacturer-recommended volume of hand rub to palm of one hand
Step 2	Rub hands together until dry, covering all surfaces of fingers and hands

Step 1: Apply product

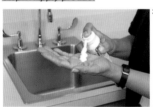

3-5

Step 2: Rub hands together until dry

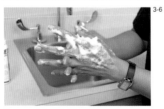

3-6

Surgical Hand Antisepsis

Surgical hand antisepsis using either an antimicrobial soap or an alcohol-based hand rub with persistent activity is recommended before donning sterile gloves when performing surgical procedures (IB).[12]

Tip: Remove rings, watches, and bracelets before starting the surgical hand scrub. Use a nail cleaner under running water to remove debris from beneath fingernails. (II) Artificial fingernails are not allowed.[12,13]

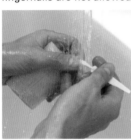

3-7

Surgical Hand Antisepsis Technique[12,13,14]	
Antimicrobial Soap	Scrub forearms and hands for the duration recommended by the manufacturer, usually 2-6 minutes. Long scrub time (e.g., 10 minutes) is unnecessary (IB)
Alcohol-Based Surgical Hand Scrub	Follow the manufacturer's instructions. Before applying alcohol solution, prewash hands and forearms with a non-antimicrobial soap, and dry hands and forearms completely. After application of the alcohol-based product as recommended, allow hands and forearms to dry thoroughly before donning sterile gloves (IB)

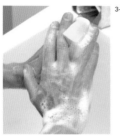

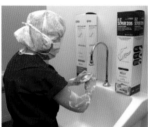

Hand Hygiene Do's and Don'ts

- **Do not** top off a partially empty soap dispenser by adding soap. This can cause bacterial contamination of soap (IA).[12]

- **Do** provide healthcare workers (HCWs) with hand creams or lotions to minimize the risk of irritant contact dermatitis associated with hand washing or antisepsis (IA).[12,13]

- **Do not** wear fingernail extensions or artificial fingernails when in direct contact with high-risk patients (IA).[12,15] Keep the tips of natural nails less than 1/4-inch long (II).[12,14] Microorganisms are harbored in the gaps of artificial fingernails and under long fingernails.[12] Also, the type and length of nails affect the efficacy of hand hygiene.[15]

- **Do** wear gloves when contact with non-intact skin, mucous membranes, and blood or other potentially infectious materials could occur (IC).[12,13,15]

- **Do** remove gloves and perform hand hygiene after caring for a patient. Do not wear the same pair of gloves for more than one patient to prevent cross-contamination, and do not wash gloves between uses with different patients (IB).[12,13,15]

- To avoid transmitting organisms from one body part to another, **DO** change gloves during patient care if moving from a contaminated body site to a clean body site (III).[12,13,15]

Patient Teaching Tip: Educate patients and their families to remind HCWs to perform hand hygiene (II).[12] Educate patients and their visitors to perform hand hygiene.

Figure References

3-1. Potter PA. Basic Nursing: Essentials for Practice. 6th ed. St Louis: Mosby; 2006.

3-2. Potter PA. Basic Nursing: Essentials for Practice. 6th ed. St Louis: Mosby; 2006.

3-3. Potter PA. Basic Nursing: Essentials for Practice. 6th ed. St Louis: Mosby; 2006.

3-4. Potter PA. Basic Nursing: Essentials for Practice. 6th ed. St Louis: Mosby; 2006.

3-5. Potter PA. Basic Nursing: Essentials for Practice. 6th ed. St Louis: Mosby; 2006.

3-6. Potter PA. Basic Nursing: Essentials for Practice. 6th ed. St Louis: Mosby; 2006.

3-7. Perry AG. Clinical Nursing Skills & Techniques. 6th ed. St Louis: Mosby; 2005.

3-8. Perry AG. Clinical Nursing Skills & Techniques. 6th ed. St Louis: Mosby; 2005.

3-9. Perry AG. Clinical Nursing Skills & Techniques. 6th ed. St Louis: Mosby; 2005.

NOTES

PERSONAL PROTECTIVE EQUIPMENT (PPE)

PERSONAL PROTECTIVE EQUIPMENT (PPE)

Types of PPE[15]	
Type of PPE	**Recommendations**
Gloves	Wear for preventing contact transmission (e.g., MRSA). Use for touching body fluid, secretions, excretions, mucous membranes, non-intact skin, blood, and contaminated items.
Surgical Mask	Use to protect HCWs from contact with large infectious droplets (>5 μm in size) and to prevent droplet transmission (e.g., influenza). Use during nursing care activities and procedures likely to generate splashes of blood, secretions, or body fluid.
Eye Protection (goggles) Face Shield	Use during nursing care activities and procedures likely to generate splashes of blood, secretions, or body fluid.
Respiratory Protector (e.g., N95 respirator)	A personal protective device worn to protect HCWs from inhalation exposure to airborne infectious droplets neuclei (<5 μm in size) and dust particles that contain infectious particles (e.g., tuberculosis, variola virus [smallpox], SARS-CoV). Must wear before entering patient's room.
Gown	Wear for preventing contact transmission. Use during nursing care and procedures when contact of clothing or exposed skin with blood, body fluid, and secretions is expected.

Sequence for Donning and Removing PPE

Always perform hand hygiene immediately before donning and after removing PPE.[12,13]

Always don your PPE before contact with patients and before entering an isolated patient's room.[15]

SEQUENCE FOR DONNING PERSONAL PROTECTIVE EQUIPMENT (PPE)

The type of PPE used will vary based on the level of precautions required; e.g., Standard and Contact, Droplet or Airborne Infection Isolation.

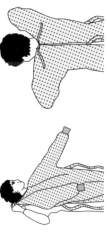

1. GOWN
   - Fully cover torso from neck to knees, arms to end of wrists, and wrap around the back
   - Fasten in back of neck and waist

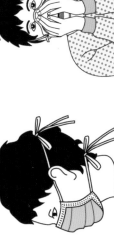

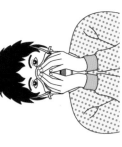

2. MASK OR RESPIRATOR

- Secure ties or elastic bands at middle of head and neck
  - Fit flexible band to nose bridge
  - Fit snug to face and below chin
  - Fit-check respirator

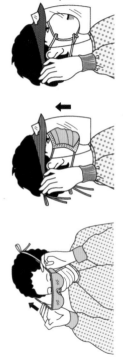

3. GOGGLES OR FACE SHIELD

- Place over face and eyes and adjust to fit

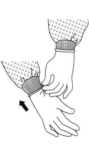

4. GLOVES

- Extend to cover wrist of isolation gown

Use Safe work practices to protect yourself and limit the spread of contamination

- Keep hands away from face
- Limit surfaces touched
- Change gloves when torn or heavily contaminated
- Perform hand hygiene

SEQUENCE FOR REMOVING PERSONAL PROTECTIVE EQUIPMENT (PPE)

Except for respirator, remove PPE at doorway or in anteroom. Remove respirator after leaving patient room and closing door.

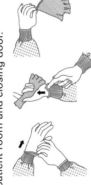

1. GLOVES
- Outside of gloves is contaminated!
- Grasp outside of glove with opposite gloved hand; peel off
- Hold removed glove in gloved hand
- Slide fingers of ungloved hand under remaining glove at wrist
- Peel glove off over first glove
- Discard gloves in waste container

Sequence for Removing PPE (continued)

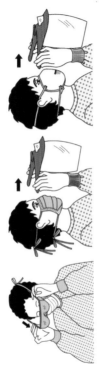

2. GOGGLES OR FACE SHIELD

- Outside of goggles or face shield is contaminated!
- To remove, handle by head band or ear pieces
- Place in designated receptacle for reprocessing or in waste container

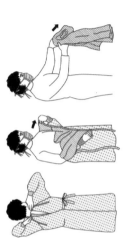

3. GOWN

- Gown front and sleeves are contaminated!
- Unfasten ties
- Pull away from neck and shoulders, touching inside of gown only
- Turn gown inside out
- Fold or roll into a bundle and discard

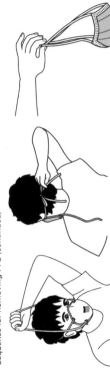

4. MASK OR RESPIRATOR

- Front of mask/respirator is contaminated — DO NOT TOUCH!
- Grasp bottom, then top ties or elastics and remove
- Discard in waste container

Perform hand hygiene immediately after removing all PPE.

Figure References

4-1. Courtesy of the Centers for Disease Control and Prevention, U.S. Department of Health and Human Services, Atlanta, Georgia.

ISOLATION PRECAUTIONS

Standard Precautions

- Standard precautions should be applied to all patients, based on the principle that all blood, body fluid, secretions, excretions, non-intact skin, and mucous membranes may contain transmissible infectious pathogens.[15]

- Hand hygiene should be performed before and after patient contact.[12]

- Healthcare providers should use PPE (gloves, surgical masks, gowns, face shields, eye protection), depending on the anticipated exposure, regardless of suspected or confirmed infection status.

- New elements of Standard Precautions from CDC Isolation Precautions Guidelines 2007[15]:

  - Respiratory Hygiene/Cough Etiquette includes:
    1. Covering the mouth/nose with a tissue when coughing/sneezing and prompt disposal of used tissues.
    2. Using surgical masks on the coughing person when tolerated and appropriate.

  - Safe Infection Practice: Use a sterile, single-use, disposable needle/syringe for each injection. Never reinsert a used needle into a multiple-dose vial or solution bag.

  - Use of surgical masks for spinal or epidural catheter insertion or injection of material into spinal or epidural spaces via lumbar procedures (e.g., myelogram, lumbar puncture, and spinal or epidural anesthesia) to prevent bacterial meningitis following myelogram and other spinal procedures due to droplet transmission of streptococcal species (a type of common oral-pharyngeal flora).

Transmission-Based Precautions[15]

- Three categories of Transmission-Based Precautions: Contact Precautions, Droplet Precautions, and Airborne Precautions. Standard Precautions should be always used in addition to Transmission-Based Precautions.

- When Standard Precautions alone cannot completely interrupt the mode of transmission, Transmission-Based Precautions should be applied.

- Transmission-Based Precautions should be applied to patients known or suspected to be infected with transmissible pathogens. (Don't wait for the culture results.)

- Some diseases have multiple modes of transmission (e.g., SARS); more than one Transmission-Based Precaution will be applied.

Contact Precautions[12,15]:

- Contact Precautions are used to prevent transmission of pathogens that are spread by direct or indirect contact with the patient, inanimate objects, or the patient's environment.

- Contact Precautions should apply to patients with excessive wound drainage, uncontrolled diarrhea, or other discharges from the body, since these may indicate an increased potential for risk of transmission and environmental contamination.

- Apply in addition to Standard Precautions.

Hand Hygiene

- Perform hand hygiene before and after each contact with a patient or patient's bedside environment/medical items.

- For *Clostridium difficile* patients, wash hands with soap and water (rather than alcohol-based hand rubs) for mechanical removal of spores from hands.

PPE

- Wear gloves and gown before entering the room, and remove gloves and gown before leaving the room.

- Remove PPE carefully, and place used PPE in the proper container to prevent environmental or self-contamination. Clean hands immediately.

Patient Placement

- Patients should be placed in a private room.

- If a private room is unavailable, place patients with the same pathogen but no other infection in the same room. Also inform the ICP for risk assessment.

- Patients should be more than 3 feet apart. Use the privacy curtain between beds to separate patients, thereby minimizing the chance for direct contact.

- If a patient must be placed in an open bed unit, visibly separate the patient's bed by a curtain.

Precaution Sign

- Post the Contact Precautions sign where clearly visible.

Visitors

- Staff shall instruct visitors on Contact Precautions.

- Clean hands before entering and leaving room.

- Wear gown and gloves when entering the room.

- Remove PPE and clean hands when leaving the room.

Patient Transport

- Notify receiving department about the patient's isolation status.

- Wounds are covered, and body fluids are contained.

- Patients should wear a clean hospital gown and clean their hands prior to leaving the room.

- Use hospital-approved disinfectant to wipe wheelchair or stretcher after transporting patients.

Medical Equipment

- When possible, dedicate equipment (e.g., stethoscope, blood pressure cuff) to single-patient use.

- Reusable patient-care equipment must be disinfected with a hospital-approved disinfectant before use on another patient.

- For *C. difficile* patients: clean equipment with a bleach-containing disinfectant solution/wipes (5000 ppm).

Room Cleaning

- For *C. difficile* patients: clean room with a bleach-containing disinfectant for environmental disinfection.

- For non-*C. difficile* patients: clean room with hospital-approved disinfectants.

Ambulation

- Ambulatory patients should wear a clean hospital gown and clean their hands prior to leaving the room.

CONTACT PRECAUTIONS *(in addition to Standard Precautions)*

VISITORS: Report to nurse before entering.

Patient Placement

Private room, if possible. Cohort if private room is not available.

Gloves

Wear gloves when entering the room. **Change** gloves after having contact with infective material that may contain high concentrations of micro-organisms (**fecal material** and **wound drainage**). **Remove** gloves before leaving patient room.

Wash

Wash hands with an **antimicrobial** agent immediately after glove removal. After glove removal and handwashing, ensure that hands do not touch potentially contaminated environmental surfaces or items in the patient's room to avoid transfer of microorganisms to other patients or environments.

Gown

Wear gown when **entering** patient room if you anticipate that your clothing will have substantial contact with the patient, environment surfaces, or items in the patient's room, or if the patient is **incontinent**, or has **diarrhea**, an **ileostomy**, a **colostomy** or **wound drainage** not contained by a dressing. **Remove** gown before leaving the patient's environment and ensure that clothing does not contact potentially contaminated environmental surfaces to avoid transfer of microorganisms to other patients or environments.

Patient Transport

Limit transport of patient to essential purposes only. During transport, ensure that precautions are maintained to minimize the risk of transmission of microorganisms to other patients and contamination of environmental surfaces and equipment.

Patient-Care Equipment

Dedicate the use of noncritical patient-care equipment to a single patient. If common equipment is used, clean and disinfect between patients.

Droplet Precautions[12,15]

Droplet precautions are used to prevent transmission of infectious agents through close respiratory or mucous-membrane contact with large-particle droplets (>5 μm in size) generated by coughing, sneezing, or talking.

- Apply in addition to Standard Precautions.

Hand Hygiene

- Perform hand hygiene before and after contact with each patient or patient's bedside environment.

PPE

- Disposable surgical mask must be worn when within 3 feet of the patient.

- Masks are single use.

Patient Placement

- Placing patients in a private room is preferred, especially if the patient exhibits excessive coughing/sneezing.

- If a private room is unavailable, place patients with the same pathogen but no other infections in the same room. Maintain spatial separation of at least 3 feet between the infected patient and other patients or visitors. Also inform the ICP for risk assessment.

Precaution Sign

- Post the Droplet Precautions sign where clearly visible.

Visitors

- Staff shall instruct visitors on Droplet Precautions.
- Clean hands before entering and leaving room.
- Visitors shall wear a surgical mask when coming within 3 feet of the patient and shall remove the mask immediately before leaving the patient's room.

Patient Transport

- Limit transport of the patient outside of the room to medical necessity only.
- If transportation is necessary, place a surgical mask on the patient.
- Notify the department receiving the patient that Droplet Precautions are necessary.

Medical Equipment

- When possible, dedicate equipment (e.g., stethoscope, blood pressure cuff) to single-patient use.
- Reusable patient-care equipment must be disinfected with the hospital-approved disinfectant before use on another patient.

Room Cleaning

- Clean room with hospital-approved disinfectants.

Ambulation

- Patients on Droplet Precautions are encouraged to stay in their rooms.

- If the patient must leave the room, a surgical mask should be worn.
- Respiratory Hygiene/Cough Etiquette should be applied.

DROPLET PRECAUTIONS *(in addition to Standard Precautions)*

VISITORS: Report to nurse before entering.

Patient Placement
Private room, if possible. Cohort or maintain spatial separation of **3 feet** from other patients or visitors if private room is not available.

Mask
Wear mask when working within **3 feet** of patient (or upon entering room).

Patient Transport
Limit transport of patient from room to essential purposes only.
Use **surgical mask** on patient during transport.

Form No. **DPR**   BREVIS CORP., 3310 S 2700 E, SLC, UT 84109   © 1996 Brevis Corp.

Airborne Precautions[12,15,17]

Airborne Precautions are used to prevent person-to-person and environmental transmission via the airborne route.

Airborne transmission occurs by disseminating either airborne droplet nuclei residue of evaporated droplets or dust particles containing the infectious agent.

Apply in addition to Standard Precautions.

Hand Hygiene

• Clean hands before entering and leaving the patient's room.

PPE

• HCWs should wear a respirator (e.g., N-95 respirator) before entering patient's room. HCWs should complete fit-testing training and know the size of respirator to wear.

• For patient's with varicella (chickenpox), disseminated herpes zoster (shingles), or measles:
  • Susceptible (nonimmune) HCWs should not be assigned to care for these patients or allowed to enter their rooms if immune HCWs are available.
  • Susceptible visitors should not visit these patients.

Room Placement

• Patient must be placed in an airborne infection isolation room (AIIR), a single-patient room equipped with a high-efficiency particulate air (HEPA) filter and ventilation system that can clean the air before the air returns to the general ventilation system. The room maintains a negative pressure relative to the surrounding area, with 6 (existing facility) or 12 (new construction/renovation) air changes per hour (ACH).

- The AIIR door should be closed when not required for entry and exit, including when the patient is out of the room for tests. Minimize unnecessary entry into the room.

- In ambulatory clinics, place the patient in an AIIR as soon as possible. If an AIIR is unavailable, place a surgical mask on the patient and place him/her in an examination room. After the patient leaves, the room should be left vacant long enough to allow for a full exchange of air, generally one hour.

Precaution Sign

- Post the Airborne Precautions sign outside the room where it is clearly visible.

Visitors

- Staff shall instruct visitors on Airborne Precautions.

- Visitors should comply with hospital Airborne Precautions policy.

- Visitors must be instructed how to wear the surgical mask correctly (cover nose and mouth entirely). Visitors do not complete fit-testing training.

Patient Transport

- Limit transportation of the patient outside of the AIIR room to only when medically necessary.

- If transport is necessary, place a surgical mask on the patient.

- Notify the department receiving the patient that Airborne Precautions are necessary.

- For patients with drainage and skin lesions associated with smallpox, varicella, or *Mycobacterium tuberculosis*, cover affected areas to prevent contact with or aerosolization of infectious agents in skin lesions.

Room Cleaning

- Standard practice: clean the room with hospital-approved disinfectant.

- The room should be vacant with the door closed for an hour after the patient leaves the room.

- If less than 1 hour has passed since the patient has left the room, anyone entering the room should wear a respirator.

Ambulation

Patient should leave room only for necessary treatment and wear surgical mask when outside of room.

Discharge

- Upon discharge, close room for 1 hour before admitting next patient.

AIRBORNE PRECAUTIONS *(in addition to Standard Precautions)*

VISITORS: Report to nurse before entering.

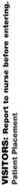

Patient Placement

Use **private room** that has:

Monitored negative air pressure,

6 to 12 air changes per hour,

Discharge of air outdoors or HEPA filtration if recirculated.

Keep room door closed and patient in room.

Respiratory Protection

Wear an **N95 respirator** when entering the room of a patient with known or suspected infectious pulmonary **tuberculosis.**

Susceptible persons should not enter the room of patients known or suspected to have **measles** (rubeola) or **varicella** (chickenpox) if other immune caregivers are available. If susceptible persons must enter, they should wear an **N95 respirator.** (Respirator or surgical mask not required if immune to measles and varicella.)

Patient Transport

Limit transport of patient from room to essential purposes only.

Use **surgical mask** on patient during transport.

Recommended Precautions for Selected Conditions[15]

Contact Precautions

- Multidrug-resistant organism (MDRO) infection or colonization, methicillin-resistant *Staphylococcus aureus* (MRSA), vancomycin-resistant enterococci (VRE), vancomycin-intermediate/resistant and vancomycin-resistant *Staphylococcus aureus* (VISA/VRSA), extended-spectrum beta-lactamases (ESBLs), multidrug-resistant *Streptococcus pneumoniae*

- Noroviruses

- Rotavirus

- *C. difficile*

- Uncontrolled diarrhea (before the culture report becomes available)

- Draining wound/abscess (before the culture report becomes available)

- Herpes simplex (disseminated or neonatal)

- Acute viral infection: enterovirus 70, Coxsackie virus A24

- Hepatitis A: only for diapered or incontinent patients

- Lice, scabies

- Poliomyelitis

- Respiratory syncytial virus (RSV) infection

- Streptococcal disease (Group A streptococcus) in major skin lesion, wound, burn: requires Droplet Precautions as well for the first 24 hours of appropriate antimicrobial therapy

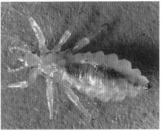
Lice have six legs and are wingless.

Droplet Precautions

- Pharyngeal diphtheria

- Pertussis (whooping cough)

- *Haemophilus influenzae* type B epiglottitis

- Seasonal influenza, pandemic influenza

- *Neisseria meningitidis* (meningococcal) meningitis, *Haemophilus influenzae* type B meningitis

- Meningococcal disease: sepsis, pneumonia, meningitis

- Mumps

- Parvovirus B19

- Rhinovirus

- Rubella (German measles)

- *Mycoplasma* pneumonia

- Adenovirus: requires Contact Precautions as well

- Streptococcus, Group A infection (besides skin lesions)

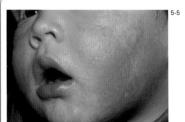

Erythema infectiosum (fifth disease, or slapped cheek). In this infection by parvovirus B19, a child will develop prominent erythema of the cheeks, aka "slapped cheeks."

Airborne Precautions

- Measles (rubeola)

- Cough, fever, and upper-lobe pulmonary infiltrate in chest x-ray (before the sputum culture report becomes available, since this may be a tuberculosis case)

- Tuberculosis (M. tuberculosis): pulmonary or laryngeal disease

- Tuberculosis (M. tuberculosis): draining wound: requires Contact Precautions as well

- Varicella zoster: requires Contact Precautions as well

- Herpes zoster (shingles): in immunocompromised patient with localized shingles or any patient with disseminated shingles. Shingles requires Contact Precautions as well

- Severe acute respiratory syndrome (SARS): requires Contact and Droplet Precautions and eye protection as well

- Avian influenza: requires Contact Precautions and eye protection as well

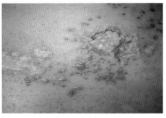
5-6

Herpes zoster. Necrotic blisters and erosions in a dermatomal pattern are seen on the trunk of this patient.

Figure References

5-1. Christensen BL. Foundations and Adult Health Nursing. 5th ed. St Louis: Mosby; 2005.

5-2. Christensen BL. Foundations and Adult Health Nursing. 5th ed. St Louis: Mosby; 2005.

5-3. Christensen BL. Foundations and Adult Health Nursing. 5th ed. St Louis: Mosby; 2005.

5-4. Christensen BL. Foundations and Adult Health Nursing. 5th ed. St Louis: Mosby; 2005.

5-5. Goldman L, Ausiello DA. Cecil Medicine: Expert Consult. 23rd ed. Philadelphia: Saunders; 2007.

5-6. Goldman L, Ausiello DA. Cecil Medicine: Expert Consult. 23rd ed. Philadelphia: Saunders; 2007.

NOTES

PREVENTION OF HEALTHCARE-ASSOCIATED INFECTIONS

PREVENTION OF HEALTHCARE-ASSOCIATED INFECTIONS

Multidrug-Resistant Organisms (MDROs)

MDROs are microorganisms, mainly bacteria, resistant to one or more classes of antibiotic agents.[18] Commonly seen MDROs include methicillin-resistant *Staphylococcus aureus* (MRSA), vancomycin-resistant enterococci (VRE), penicillin-resistant *Streptococcus pneumoniae* (PRSP), and extended-spectrum beta-lactamases (ESBLs) producing gram-negative bacilli.

Healthcare-associated MDRO infections are on the rise because antibiotics are frequently prescribed in hospitals. Hospitalized patients are often immunocompromised due to underlying diseases or treatments, making them vulnerable to acquiring MDRO infections with opportunistic or virulent pathogens.

The effects of MDROs range from asymptomatic colonization (carrier) to potentially life-threatening infections such as sepsis and pneumonia. Therapeutic options for treating MDRO infections are very limited.

Both MDRO colonization and infection are transmissible.

MDRO infections increase length of hospital stay, medical costs, mortality, and chance of admission to the ICU. MDRO prevention and control has become a top national priority in all healthcare settings.

There are several risk factors for both MDRO colonization and infection.[19]

Risk Factors for Developing MDRO Colonization and Infection

Categories	Risk Factors
Patient Characteristics	Advanced age
	Severity of illness
	Preexisting disease or conditions: • Diabetes mellitus • Chronic renal disease • Peripheral vascular disease • Weakened immune system: oncology patients and organ transplant patients
Antibiotic Therapy	Exposure to antimicrobial treatment in previous 2 weeks
Invasive Catheters	Presence of invasive catheterization or urinary catheter
Contact with Healthcare Facilities	• Multiple hospitalizations • Repeatedly accessing healthcare setting (e.g., patients needing dialysis three times per week)
Previous Colonization with MDROs	Previous colonization by MDRO: previous VRE rectal colonization is a risk factor for developing VRE urinary tract infection.
Skin Condition	• Presence of wounds • Decubitus ulcers • Skin lesions • Dermatitis • Burns

6-1

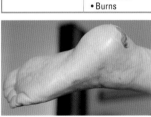

Decubitus ulcer. Skin forms craterlike lesions when blood supply is diminished. Integrity of skin tissue cannot be maintained in the area of reduced blood flow.

Recommendations for Prevention of Transmission of Healthcare-Associated MDROs[18,19,20]

CDC Guidelines: Control Measures to Prevent Transmission of MDROs

Administrative Measures:

1. Provide administrative support and make control and prevention of MDROs an institutional patient-safety priority (IB).[18,20]
2. Ensure that a multidisciplinary process is in place to monitor and improve HCWs' compliance with recommended practices for Standard Precautions and Contact Precautions (IB).[18,20]
3. Implement systems to identify patients colonized or infected with MDROs and to notify receiving healthcare facilities prior to transferring such patients (IB).[18,20]

Education and Training:

1. Educate and train HCWs on risks and prevention of transmission of MDROs at orientation and through periodic educational updates (IB).[18,20]

Judicious Antimicrobial Usage:

1. Implement a multidisciplinary process to review antibiotic use and institutional susceptibility patterns (antibiograms) (IB).[18,20]

Surveillance:

1. In all healthcare organizations, establish systems to ensure that clinical microbiology laboratories (in-house and outsourced) promptly notify ICP or a designee when a novel resistance pattern for that facility is detected (IB).[18,19,20]
2. Monitor the frequency of target MDROs in the facility to determine if MDRO rates are decreasing and if additional interventions are needed (IA).[18,19,20]

3. Identify readmission cases with previous history of MDRO.[19]

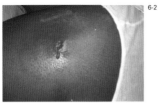

6-2

This 2005 photograph depicted a cutaneous abscess located on the hip of a prison inmate, which had begun to spontaneously drain, releasing its purulent contents. The abscess was caused by methicillin-resistant *Staphylococcus aureus* bacteria, referred to by the acronym MRSA.

Infection Control Precautions:

1. Always follow Standard Precautions during patient care (IB).[1,18,19,20]

2. Use masks or face shields when performing procedures that might result in splashing (e.g., intubation, wound irrigation, oral suctioning); when caring for patients with the potential for projectile secretions (e.g., open tracheostomies); and when there is evidence of transmission from heavily colonized sources (e.g., burn wounds) (IB).[1,18,19,20]

3. In acute-care facilities, routinely employ Contact Precautions for all patients with target MDROs and for patients previously identified as being colonized with target MDROs (IB).[1,18,19,20]

4. In ambulatory and home care settings, use Standard Precautions for patients infected or colonized with target MDROs, using gowns and gloves when in contact with uncontrolled secretions, draining wounds, pressure ulcers, stool incontinence, and ostomy bags and tubes (II).[18,19,20]

5. Limit the amount of reusable medical equipment brought into the room/home of patients infected or colonized with MDROs. Whenever possible, leave equipment in the room/home until the patient is discharged (II).[18,19,20] After patient is discharged, clean reusable medical equipment with hospital-approved disinfectant.

6. If noncritical medical equipment (e.g., stethoscopes) cannot remain in the room/home of patient, clean items with hospital-approved disinfectant before removing them from the room/home, or place items in a plastic bag for transport to another site for cleaning and disinfection (II).[18,20]

7. When available, assign priority for single-patient rooms to patients with known or suspected MDRO infection or colonization, giving priority to those having conditions that may facilitate transmission (e.g., uncontained excretions or secretions) (IB).[1,18,20]

8. Place patients with the same MDRO in the same room or patient-care area when single-patient rooms are unavailable (IB).[1,18,19,20]

BODY SUBSTANCE ISOLATION IS FOR ALL PATIENT CARE	BODY SUBSTANCES INCLUDE ORAL SECRETIONS, BLOOD, URINE AND FECES, WOUND OR OTHER DRAINAGE.

Wash hands.

Wear gloves when likely to touch body substances, mucous membranes or nonintact skin.

Wear mask/eye protection when likely to be splashed.

Wear plastic apron when clothing is likely to be soiled.

Place intact needle/syringe units and sharps in designated disposal container. **Do not** break or bend needles.

© 1987 San Diego Forms

Environmental Decontamination:

1. Clean and disinfect high-touch surfaces and equipment that may be contaminated with pathogens (e.g., bedrails, bedside commodes, bathroom fixtures in the patient's room, doorknobs) more frequently than minimal-touch surfaces (e.g., horizontal surfaces in waiting rooms) (IB).[18,20]

2. Dedicate noncritical patient-care items for use on individual patients known to be infected or colonized with MDROs (IB).[18,19,20]

3. Continue to monitor the occurrence of target MDRO infection and colonization after implementing additional interventions, implementing further interventions to reduce MDRO transmission if rates do not decrease (IB).[18,20]

Decolonization:

1. Decolonization therapy should be applied on a case-by-case basis, since decolonization therapy is not 100% effective and carries a risk of developing resistance to agents.[19]

2. When decolonization for MRSA is applied, perform susceptibility testing for the decolonizing agent against the target organism in the individual. Monitor susceptibility to detect emergence of resistance to the decolonizing agent (IB).[18,20]

Intravascular Catheter-Associated Bloodstream Infections (CA-BSI)

Approximately 70% to 90% of bloodstream infections (BSI) occur in patients with a central venous catheter (CVC). CA-BSI has an attributable mortality rate of 18%.[21,22,23,24,25]

The Institute for Healthcare Improvement (IHI) recommended five key components for reducing the incidence of CA-BSI: (1) hand hygiene, (2) subclavian vein placement as the preferred site, (3) chlorhexidine skin preparation, (4) full-barrier precautions during central venous catheter insertion, and (5) daily review of central line necessity.[21,23] These five components are based on best practice guidelines and comply with CDC's Guidelines for the Prevention of Intravascular Catheter-Related Infections for patients undergoing insertion of central venous catheters. Together, these are referred to as the "central line bundle." Here, *bundle* means a group of evidence-based interventions.[21,23]

The five species of bacteria most frequently isolated from blood cultures are coagulase-negative staphylococci, *S. aureus*, *Enterococcus faecalis*, *Escherichia coli*, and *Klebsiella pneumoniae*.[21]

Risk Factors for Central Venous Catheter–Associated Bloodstream Infection (CA-BSI)[21,22,23,24,25]	
Categories	**Risk Factors**
Patient Characteristics	Many specific patients are vulnerable to CA-BSI: • The elderly • Neonates • Patients with severe illness • Burn patients • Neutropenia/immunodeficiency patients • Dialysis patients
Type of Central Venous Catheter (CVC)	• Patients with multilumen CVCs have a higher CA-BSI rate than those with single-lumen catheters.[21]
Location of Central Venous Catheter	• Patients with CVCs in the femoral vein show the highest incidence of CA-BSI. Next are patients with CVCs in the internal jugular. The subclavian vein has the lowest rate of BSI. The subclavian vein is therefore the pre-

	ferred site when inserting non-tunneled CVCs in adults if there is no medical contraindication.[21,22,23,24]
Type of IV Fluid Infusion	• CVCs used to administer TPN and/or lipids are associated with increased incidence of BSI. These BSIs are polymicrobial and fungi infections.[21] • CVCs used to administer blood-product transfusions have a higher rate of BSI.[21] • To protect patients: [21] 1. Before accessing the IV, antiseptic technique should be applied. 2. Before accessing the injection system, clean the injection ports with 70% alcohol or an iodophor, and allow to air dry. 3. After infusion, catheter should be flushed with sterile, preservative-free normal saline.
Other Risk Factors	• Inexperience of the physician inserting the CVC[21,22,23] • Low nurse/patient ratio[21,22,23]

Recommendations for Prevention of Intravascular Catheter-Associated Bloodstream Infections (CA-BSI)[21,22,23]

CDC Guidelines: Control Measures to Prevent Intravascular Catheter-Associated BSI

Education and Training:

1. HCWs should be provided periodic in-service regarding indications of intravenous catheterization, proper procedure of insertion and care of central venous catheters, and prevention of BSI.

Hand Hygiene[12]:

1. Perform proper hand hygiene either by washing hands with antimicrobial soap and water or with waterless alcohol-based hand rubs:
   - before and after palpating catheter insertion sites (IA)[22,23]
   - before and after inserting, replacing, accessing, repairing, or dressing an intravascular catheter (IA)[22,23]
2. Wearing gloves does not replace the necessity for hand hygiene (IA).[22]

Replacement of Intravascular Catheters:

1. Promptly remove intravascular catheters that are no longer essential (IA).[22,23]
2. Do not routinely change CVCs, peripherally inserted central catheters (PICCs), hemodialysis catheters, or pulmonary artery catheters solely to reduce catheter-related infections (IB).[22]
3. Do not remove CVCs or PICCs on the basis of fever alone. Use clinical judgment regarding the appropriateness of removing the catheter if infection is evidenced elsewhere or if a noninfectious cause of fever is suspected (II).[22]
4. Replace short-term CVCs if purulence is noted at the insertion site, indicating infection (IB).[21,22]
5. Do not use guidewire techniques for replacing catheters in patients with suspected catheter-related infection (IB).[22]
6. If there is no evidence of infection, use guidewire exchange to replace malfunctioning non-tunneled catheters (IB).[22]

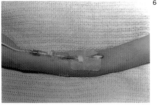

6-4

Peripheral intravenous catheter for parenteral nutrition. There has recently been a move back to appropriate peripheral intravenous cannulae for parenteral nutrition. The risk of serious complications may be lower than with central catheterization.

Catheter Insertion Site Dressing Regimens:

1. Cover the catheter site with either sterile gauze or sterile, transparent, semipermeable dressing (IA).[22]

2. Gauze dressing is preferable if the patient is diaphoretic or if the site is oozing or bleeding (II).[22]

3. If the catheter-site dressing becomes loosened, damp, or visibly soiled, replace it (IB).[22]

4. Except when using dialysis catheters, do not use topical antibiotic cream or ointment on insertion sites. These may promote antimicrobial resistance and fungal infections (IA).[22]

5. Do not routinely administer antimicrobial prophylaxis before insertion or during use of an intravascular catheter to prevent catheter colonization or infection (IA).[22]

6. Employ aseptic technique, including use of a sterile gown, sterile gloves, cap, mask, and large sterile drape, for insertion of CVCs and PICCs or guidewire exchange (IA).[22,23]

7. Protect pulmonary artery catheters with a sterile sleeve during insertion (IB).[22]

Catheter-Site Care:

1. Disinfect clean skin with an appropriate antiseptic before inserting catheters and while changing dressings. A 2% chlorhexidine-based preparation is preferred, but an iodophor, tincture of iodine, or 70% alcohol agent can be used (IA).[22]

2. Evidence suggests that antiseptic 2% chlorhexidine gluconate in 70% isopropyl alcohol provides better antisepsis than iodine. To prepare the insertion site, press the applicator against the insertion site and apply the antiseptic solution using a back-and-forth friction scrub for at least 30 seconds.[23]

3. No recommendation can be made for using chlorhexidine-based skin antisepsis on patients under 2 months of age.[22]

4. Allow the antiseptic on the insertion site to air dry before inserting the catheter. Antiseptic solution should remain on the skin for at least 2 minutes, longer if not yet dry before insertion. Never wipe or blot to dry (IB).[22]

Replacement of Administration IV Tubing and Needleless Systems:

1. Unless catheter-related infection is documented or suspected, do not replace administration IV tubing, including add-on devices and secondary sets, more frequently than at 72-hour intervals (IA).[22]

2. Tubing used to administer blood, blood products, or lipid emulsions should be replaced within 24 hours of beginning the infusion (IB).[22] It is unnecessary to replace IV infusion tubing more frequently than every 72 hours if the solution contains only dextrose and amino acids (II).[22]

3. Tubing used to administer propofol infusions should be replaced every 6 to 12 hours, depending on use and the manufacturer's recommendation (IA).[22]

4. Change needleless intravascular caps no more frequently than every 72 hours or according to the recommendation of the manufacturer (II).[22]

5. Wipe the access port with an appropriate antiseptic and access the port only with sterile devices to minimize contamination risk (IB). Use 70% alcohol or an iodophor to clean injection ports before accessing the system (IA).[22]

6. Infusion of lipid-containing solutions (e.g., 3-in-1 solutions) should be completed within 24 hours of hanging the solution (IB).[22]

7. Infusion of lipid emulsions alone should be completed within 12 hours of hanging the emulsion. If more time is required due to volume considerations, complete the infusion within 24 hours (IB).[22]

8. Infusions of blood or other blood products should be completed within 4 hours of hanging the blood (II).[22]

9. When not in use, cap all stopcocks (IB).[22]

Preparation and Quality Control of IV Admixtures:

1. Do not use a parenteral fluid container if the expiration date has passed, if it is cloudy, or if it has visible cracks, leaks, or particulate matter (IB).[22]

2. After using single-use vials, do not combine the leftover contents for later use (IA).[22]

3. Use 70% alcohol to clean the access diaphragms of multidose vials before inserting devices (IA).[22]

4. Access a multidose vial using a sterile device, and avoid touch contamination before penetrating its access diaphragm (IA).[22]

Catheter-Associated Urinary Tract Infection (UTI)

Hospital-acquired urinary tract infections make up 40% of all HAIs. Eighty percent of hospital-acquired UTIs are due to use of indwelling urethral catheters. Indwelling catheters are used in 12% to 16% of hospital inpatients.[26]

Urinary tract infections can cause systemic and local morbidity and secondary bloodstream infection. They can also provide a reservoir for drug-resistant organisms. As a result, mortality, medical costs, and use of antibiotics are increased, and hospital stays are prolonged.

Common pathogens causing UTI are[27,28]:

- Gram-negative bacilli: E. coli, Klebsiella spp., Proteus spp., Pseudomonas spp., or Serratia spp.

- Gram-positive cocci: enterococci, staphylococci

- Candida/Yeasts

Risk Factors for Developing Urinary Tract Infection[27,28,29]

Categories	Risk Factors
Patient Characteristics	• Postpartum status • Advanced age • Severe underlying illness • Renal insufficiency, high blood creatinine level • Diabetes mellitus/poor glucose control • Frequent sexual activity
Gender	• Females more susceptible than males • Previous history of UTI in female patients • Urinary incontinence in females • Recent genitourinary surgery in females
Urinary Catheter	• Indwelling urinary catheters • Contamination during catheter insertion • Unnecessary urinary catheterization • Errors in caring for urinary catheters

Recommendations for Prevention of Urinary Tract Infection[27,28,29]

CDC Guidelines: Control Measures to Prevent Catheter-Associated Urinary Tract Infection

Education and Training

1. HCWs should be provided periodic in-service regarding indications of urinary catheterization, proper procedure for insertion and care of urinary catheters, and prevention of UTI.

Hand Hygiene[12]:

1. Hand hygiene should be performed before and after any manipulation of the catheter or catheter site.[28]

Catheter Insertion[27,28,29]:

1. Insert urinary catheters only when necessary, and keep them in place only as long as necessary. Urinary catheters should not be used for the convenience of HCWs.
2. Catheters should be inserted and manipulated by trained HCWs, family members, or patients.
3. Use sterile equipment and aseptic technique when inserting catheters.
4. Use gloves, sponges, drape, appropriate antiseptic solution for periurethral cleaning, and a single-use packet of lubricant jelly for insertion.
5. Use as small a catheter as possible, consistent with good drainage, to minimize trauma to the urethra.

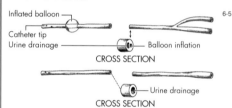

Indwelling and straight urinary catheters.

Catheter Care and Maintenance[27,28,29]:

1. After insertion, indwelling catheters should be properly secured with a catheter-securing device to eliminate tension on the balloon and prevent movement and urethral traction.[28]
2. Urinary flow should remain unobstructed. This may be accomplished by keeping the collection bag below the level of the bladder at all times, ensuring that the catheter tube remains free from kinking, and regularly emptying the collection bag, using a different container for each patient and ensuring

that the drainage spigot does not come into direct contact with the collecting container.

3. To prevent transmission of organisms, Standard Precautions should be used when manipulating urine collection bags.

4. Daily meatal care with antiseptic solutions has not been shown to reduce catheter-associated UTI; routine hygiene is recommended.

Closed Drainage System:

1. A sterile, closed drainage system should be maintained.[26]

2. Do not disconnect the catheter and drainage tube unless the catheter requires irrigation.[26]

3. Avoid irrigation unless obstruction is present or anticipated. Disinfect the catheter/tubing junction before disconnection.[29]

4. The collecting urinary bag should be replaced if disconnection, break in aseptic technique, or leakage occurs. The catheter/tubing junction should be disinfected with disinfectant and with use of aseptic technique.[28,29]

Specimen Collection[29]:

1. To collect small volumes of fresh urine, disinfect the distal sampling port of the catheter, then aspirate the urine with a sterile needle and syringe.

2. Obtain larger volumes of urine aseptically from the drainage bag.

Alternative Methods[27,28]:

1. Based on the patient's condition, alternative methods of urinary drainage may be utilized:

   Condom catheter drainage

   Suprapubic catheterization

   Intermittent urethral catheterization can be a useful alternative to indwelling urethral catheterization.

Approaches that Are Not Recommended to Prevent Urinary Catheter-Associated UTI[47]

1. Continuous bladder irrigation with antimicrobials as a routine infection prevention measure
2. Screening for asymptomatic bacteruria in catheterized patients
3. Treating asymptomatic bacteruria in catheterized patients, except prior to invasive urologic procedures
4. Changing indwelling catheters at arbitrary fixed intervals

Surgical-Site Infections (SSIs)

The risk of developing (SSIs) is closely associated with the degree of microbial contamination of an incision site at the time of surgery. The pathogens causing SSI are primarily endogenous flora from the patient's skin, mucous membranes, or hollow organs.[30,32]

The risk of developing SSI is determined by four clinical variables: inoculum of bacteria, virulence of microorganisms, adjutants in the microenvironment, and impaired host defenses.[30] Some patients are more susceptible to SSI, depending on risk factors.

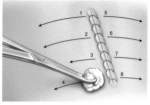

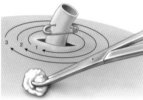

Cleaning a surgical wound. *A,* Start at the incision and clean outward. *B,* Start at the drain site and clean around the drain in a circular fashion. Use a new, clean sterile swab for each stroke to prevent contamination of the wound.

Risk Factors for Developing Surgical-Site Infections[30-32]

Patient-Related Risk Factors:

• Diabetes mellitus, poor glucose control

• Nicotine use, cigarette smoking

• Systemic steroid usage

• Malnutrition

• Advanced age

• Prolonged preoperative hospital stay

• Preoperative transfusion

• Preexisting infection or colonization at a remote body site (e.g., MRSA colonized in nares)

- Obesity
- Altered immune response: patient receiving immunosuppressant
- Higher wound classification: a patient with dirty-infected wounds (Class IV) has higher risk for developing SSI than a patient with a clean wound (Class I).

Operation-Related Risk Factors:

- Insufficient duration of surgical scrub
- Improper preoperative skin preparation
- Duration of surgery (the longer the surgery time, the higher the SSI rate)
- Pre-surgery hair shaving
- Inadequate operating room ventilation
- Inadequate sterilization of instruments
- Foreign material in the surgical site
- Surgical technique: poor hemostasis, failure to obliterate dead space, tissue trauma
- Breaking sterile technique during surgery

According to the National Nosocomial Infections Surveillance (NNIS), wound class is the CDC adaptation of the American College of Surgeons' wound classification schema. Wound classification is a predictor of SSI and is based on factors contributing to the possibility of developing SSI. Wounds are divided into four classifications: clean, clean-contaminated, contaminated, and dirty-infected wounds.

Wound Classifications, Explanations, and Surgical Procedures[30,31]

Clean Wound (Class I)

Explanation

- A noninfected surgical site having no inflammation

- Respiratory, alimentary, genital, or uninfected urinary tracts are not entered

- Surgical wound is primarily closed and drained with closed drainage

Surgical Procedures

- C-section

- Carpal tunnel repair

- Total hip replacement

Clean-Contaminated Wound (Class II)

Explanation

- A surgical site where the respiratory, alimentary, genital, or urinary tracts are entered under controlled conditions and without unusual contamination

- Surgeries involving the biliary tract, appendix, vagina, and oropharynx included in this category

Surgical Procedures

- Cholecystectomy

- Cystoscopy

- Intestinal resection

Contaminated Wound (Class III)

Explanation

- An open, fresh, accidental wound

- Operations with major breaks in sterile technique (e.g., open cardiac massage)

- Gross spillage from the gastrointestinal tract and incisions in which acute, nonpurulent inflammation is encountered included in this category

Surgical Procedures

- Gunshot

- Rectal procedure

Dirty-Infected Wound (Class IV)

Explanation

- Old traumatic wounds with retained devitalized tissue and those that involve existing clinical infection or perforated viscera

- This definition suggests that the organisms causing postoperative infection were present in the surgical site.

Surgical Procedures

- Amputation of a gangrenous limb

- Appendectomy for ruptured appendix

The most common isolated pathogens causing SSI are *S. aureus*, coagulase-negative staphylococci, *Enterococcus* spp, and *E. coli*.[31]

- *S. aureus* and coagulase-negative staphylococci are the two most common pathogens, isolated largely from clean surgical procedures.

- In recent years, more surgical sites are infected with MDROs, both gram-positive and gram-negative.

- If surgeries enter the respiratory, gastrointestinal, or gynecologic tracts, pathogens are polymicrobic with both aerobic and anaerobic bacteria.

The CDC's NNIS system has developed standardized surveillance criteria divided into three types: type of SSI, tissues involved, and clinical presentation.

The three types of SSI are:

1. Superficial incisional SSI

    a. Occurs within 30 days after the operation

    b. Tissue involves only skin or subcutaneous tissue of the incision

    c. Clinical presentations: At least one of the following:

        (i) Purulent drainage

        (ii) Organisms isolated from fluid or tissue in incision

        (iii) At least one of the following: erythema, pain/tenderness, localized swelling, or heat in superficial incision

2. Deep incisional SSI

    a. Occurs within 30 days after the operation, *or*

    b. Occurs within 1 year if implant is in place

    c. Tissue involves deep soft tissues of the incision (e.g., fascial and/or muscle layers)

d. Clinical presentations: At least one of the following:

  (i) Purulent drainage from a deep incision with no organ/space component involvement

  (ii) A deep incision ruptures or is deliberately opened by a surgeon due to infection

  (iii) An abscess or other evidence of infection involving a deep incision is found

3. Organ/space SSI

   a. Occurs within 30 days after the operation, **or**

   b. Occurs within 1 year if implant is in place

   c. Tissue involves any part of the anatomy structure that was not opened or manipulated during the surgery

   d. Clinical presentations: At least one of the following:

     (i) Purulent drainage from a drain placed into the organ/space

     (ii) Organisms isolated from culture of fluid or tissue in the organ/space

     (iii) An abscess or other evidence of infection involving the organ/space is found

SSI can be prevented by administering antimicrobial prophylaxis, complying with surgical scrub, using surgical barriers, and improving surgical technique, operating room ventilation, and sterilization methods.

Measures to Prevent Surgical-Site Infection[31]

Preparation of the Patient:

1. Identify and treat infections remote to the surgical site before elective operations. Postpone elective operations on patients until the infection has resolved. (IA)
2. Do not routinely remove hair before surgery unless the hair is at or around the incision site and interferes with the operation. (IA)
3. If hair must be removed, remove it immediately before the operation with electric clippers. (IA)
4. Adequately control serum blood glucose levels in diabetic patients. (IB)
5. Encourage cessation of tobacco product use. Instruct patients to abstain from tobacco consumption for at least 30 days before elective surgery. (IB)
6. Require patients to shower or bathe with an antiseptic agent on the night before surgery. (IB)
7. Wash and clean around the incision site to remove gross contamination before performing antiseptic skin preparation. (IB)
8. Use an appropriate antiseptic agent for skin preparation. (IB)
9. Perform pre-surgery antiseptic skin preparation in concentric circles moving from the center to the periphery. Prepare an area large enough to cover extensions of the incision, new incisions, and drain sites. (II)

Hand/Forearm Antisepsis for Surgical Team Members:

1. Keep nails short; no artificial nails are allowed. (IB)
2. Perform a preoperative surgical scrub for at least 2 to 5 minutes with a hospital-approved

antiseptic. Scrub hands and forearms up to the elbows. (IB)

3. After performing a surgical scrub, keep hands up and away from the body (elbows in flexed position) so that water runs from the tips of the fingers toward the elbows. Dry hands with a sterile towel, and put on a sterile gown and gloves. (IB)

4. Clean underneath each fingernail prior to performing the first surgical scrub of the day. (II)

5. Do not wear hand or arm jewelry. (II)

Surgical Attire and Drapes:

1. Wear a surgical mask that fully covers the mouth and nose when entering the operating room if an operation is about to begin, is already underway, or if sterile instruments are exposed. Wear the mask throughout the operation. (IB)

2. Wear a cap or hood to fully cover hair on the head and face when entering the operating room. (IB)

3. Scrubbed surgical members must put on sterile gloves after putting on a sterile gown. (IB)

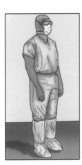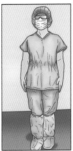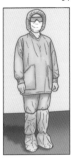

Appropriate surgical attire. *A,* When a two-piece scrub suit is worn, loose-fitting scrub tops should be tucked into pants. *B,* Tunic tops that fit close to the body may be worn outside of pants. *C,* Nonscrubbed personnel should wear long-sleeved jackets that are buttoned or snapped closed.

Antimicrobial Prophylaxis:

1. Initial doses of prophylactic antimicrobial agent should be administered through the IV route. The initial dose should be timed so that a bactericidal concentration of the drug is present in tissues and serum when the incision is first made. Therapeutic levels of the agent should be maintained in tissues and serum during the surgery and until a few hours after closing the incision. (IA)

2. Before elective colorectal surgery, in addition to the above, the colon should be prepared using enemas, and non-absorbable oral antimicrobial agents should be administered on the day before surgery. (IA)

3. For cesarean section, the prophylactic antimicrobial agent should be administered immediately after clamping the umbilical cord. (IA)

Intraoperative Ventilation:

1. Maintain positive-pressure ventilation in the operating room with respect to the corridors and adjacent areas. (IB)
2. Maintain a minimum of 15 air changes per hour, of which at least 3 should be fresh air. (IB)
3. Filter all air, recirculated and fresh, through the appropriate filters. (IB)
4. Air should be introduced from the ceiling, and should exit near the floor. (IB)
5. Keep operating room doors closed except as needed for passage of equipment, personnel, and the patient. (IB)
6. Limit the number of personnel entering the operating room. (II)

Environmental Disinfection:

1. When visible soiling or contamination of surfaces or equipment with blood or other body fluids occurs, use disinfectant to clean the affected areas before the next operation. (IB)

Sterilization of Surgical Instruments:

1. Sterilize all surgical instruments. (IB)
2. Perform flash sterilization only for patient-care items that will be used immediately. Do not use flash sterilization for reasons of convenience, as an alternative to purchasing additional instrument sets, or to save time. (IB)

Postoperative Incision Care:

1. Surgical site should be protected with a sterile dressing for 24 to 48 hours after surgery. (IB)
2. Wash hands before and after dressing changes and any contact with the surgical site. (IB)

Healthcare-Associated Pneumonia

Healthcare-associated pneumonia (HCAP), ventilator-associated pneumonia (VAP), and hospital-acquired pneumonia (HAP) remain the key causes of mortality, morbidity, prolonged hospital stay, and prolonged ventilator usage.

Introduced as a new category of pneumonia by The American Thoracic Society and the Infectious Diseases Society of America in 2005, HCAP specifically refers to pneumonia acquired as a result of recent close contact with the healthcare system. Since more patients are receiving medical treatment (e.g., dialysis, wound care, chemotherapy) outside the hospital in clinics or other facilities, the HCAP category can reflect healthcare-associated pneumonia occurring in healthcare settings other than acute-care hospitals.[33]

Categories of Pneumonia[33]	
Category	**Definition**
Healthcare-associated pneumonia (HCAP)	Pneumonia occurring in a patient who: • Was admitted to an acute care hospital more than 2 days in the 90 days prior to the infection • Resided in a long-term-care facility or nursing home • Received wound care, chemotherapy, or intravenous antibiotic therapy within 30 days of the current infection • Attended a hospital or hemodialysis clinic
Ventilator-associated pneumonia (VAP)	Pneumonia occurring more than 48 hours after endotracheal intubation on a ventilator
Hospital-acquired pneumonia (HAP)	Pneumonia occurring 48 hours or more after admission, provided there were no signs or symptoms present upon admission

Patients with HCAP are at greater risk for colonization and infection with MDROs. Infections with MDR pathogens require different empiric antibiotic therapy. To avoid initiation of inappropriate antibiotic therapy that may result in poorer patient outcomes, new principles for HCAP management were published in the American Thoracic Society and the Infectious Diseases Society of America Guidelines in 2005.

Risk Factors for Developing Healthcare-Acquired Pneumonia[33,35]

Patient Characteristic Risk Factors

- Advanced age

- Severity of underlying illness

- Being immunocompromised

- History of pulmonary diseases (COPD, emphysema)

- History of smoking

- History of dysphagia

- Having risk of aspiration (impaired airway reflexes, nasogastric tube feeding, difficulty clearing mucus in throat)

- Depressed level of consciousness

Medical Intervention Risk Factors

- Having been admitted to an intensive care unit

- Having been intubated

- Presence of a tracheostomy

- Having been on mechanically assisted ventilation

- Having been admitted to hospital greater than 48 hours

Quality Control/Patient Safety Risk Factors

- Contaminated respiratory devices/equipment (ventilator circuits, aerosols, humidifier fluid, reservoir bags)

- Inadequately sterilized anesthesia devices/equipment (face masks, of CO_2 analyzer probes)

- Inadequately sterilized laryngoscope blades

- Inadequate intra-cuff pressure

- Accidental extubation

- Failure to elevate the head of the bed

6-8

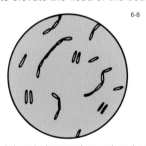

Bacilli are rod-shaped microorganisms and are the major gram-negative organisms responsible for pneumonia.

How Does Healthcare-Acquired Pneumonia Spread?[35]

Three Routes of Healthcare-Acquired Pulmonary Infection	
Via mechanical ventilator	Pathogen enters the pulmonary system through inadequately sterilized circuits or aerosol devices
Via aspiration	Aspiration of oropharyngeal organisms is the most common route of infection
Via hand-to-hand contact	The pathogen causing pneumonia can spread from patient to patient on contaminated hands of healthcare providers

Control Measures to Prevent Healthcare-Acquired Pneumonia[33,34]

Education:

• Provide education to HCWs about epidemiology and infection control procedures for preventing healthcare-associated pneumonia. Enhance their competency, and involve them in implementing interventions to prevent healthcare acquired pneumonia using performance-improvement tools and techniques. (IA)

Surveillance:

• Conduct surveillance for healthcare-associated pneumonia in intensive care unit patients to determine trends and help identify outbreaks and other potential infection control problems. Pneumonia rates should be monitored, and prevention should be implemented. Data should be returned to appropriate healthcare personnel. (IB)

Prevention of Transmission of Pathogens

Sterilization and Disinfection:

- Always thoroughly clean all equipment before sterilization or disinfection. (IA)

- Use steam sterilization or high-level disinfection by wet heat pasteurization at >158°F (>70°C) for 30 minutes for reprocessing semicritical equipment items that come into direct or indirect contact with mucous membranes of the lower respiratory tract and are not sensitive to heat and moisture.

- If semicritical equipment or devices are heat- or moisture-sensitive, use low-temperature sterilization methods. After disinfection, proceed with appropriate rinsing, drying, and packaging, taking care not to contaminate the disinfected items in the process. (IA)

- Change the circuit (ventilator tubing, exhalation valve, and the attached humidifier) only when visibly soiled or malfunctioning. Do not change routinely. (IA)

- Fill bubbling humidifiers with sterile water (not nonsterile distilled water). (II)

- Use sterile fluid for nebulization, and be certain to follow aseptic technique when filling the nebulizer. (IA)

Standard Precautions:

- Decontaminate hands with soap and water (if hands are visibly soiled) or with alcohol-based hand rub before and after contact with patients, performing procedures, or handling devices. (IA)

- Wear gloves for handling respiratory secretions or objects contaminated with respiratory secretions of any patient. (IB)

- Perform hand hygiene after removing gloves. (IA)

- Change gloves and decontaminate hands between contacts with different patients, after contact with respiratory secretions or objects contaminated with respiratory secretions from one patient before contact with a second patient, and before contact with a patient's respiratory tract or respiratory device following contact with a contaminated body site. (IA).

- When changing a tracheostomy tube, wear a gown, use aseptic technique, and replace the tube with one that has undergone sterilization or high-level disinfection. (IB)

- To prevent transmission of organisms, Standard Precautions should be used when providing breathing treatment, suctioning, and manipulating tracheostomy tubes.

Prevention of Aspiration:

- If there is no medical contraindication, elevate the head of the bed at an angle of 30 to 45 degrees for patients at high risk for aspiration. (II)

- If there is no contraindication, perform orotracheal instead of nasotracheal intubation on patients. (IB)

- Ensure that secretions are cleared from above the endotracheal tube cuff before moving the tube or deflating the cuff in preparation for tube removal. (II)

Prevention of Oropharyngeal Colonization:

- Clean and decontaminate oropharyngeal colonization with an antiseptic agent by implementing comprehensive oral-hygiene care for patients at high risk for healthcare-associated pneumonia. (II)

• Prior to surgery, use an oral chlorhexidine gluconate (0.12%) rinse for adult patients who undergo cardiac surgery. (II)

Prevention of Postoperative Pneumonia:

• If there is no medical contraindication, encourage postoperative patients to take deep breaths and ambulate. (IB)

• Use incentive spirometry on postoperative patients at high risk for pneumonia. (IB)

Pneumococcal Vaccination: Vaccinate Patients at High Risk for Severe Pneumococcal Infections: (Adapted from Guidelines for Preventing Healthcare-Associated Pneumonia, 2003)

• Administer the 23-valent pneumococcal polysaccharide vaccine to:

   a. patients aged ≥65 years

   b. patients aged between 5 to 64 years who have chronic cardiovascular disease (e.g., congestive heart failure or cardiomyopathy), chronic pulmonary disease (e.g., COPD or emphysema), diabetes mellitus, alcoholism, chronic liver disease, or cerebrospinal fluid (CSF) leaks

   c. patients aged between 5 to 64 years who have functional or anatomic asplenia

   d. patients aged between 5 to 64 years who are living in special environments or social settings

e. immunocompromised patients aged ≥5 years with HIV infection, leukemia, lymphoma, Hodgkin's disease, multiple myeloma, generalized malignancy, chronic renal failure, nephrotic syndrome, or other conditions associated with immunosuppression (e.g., receipt of solid-organ transplant, immunosuppressive therapy, chemotherapy, or long-term systemic corticosteroid treatment)

f. patients in long-term-care facilities (IA)

- Administer the 7-valent pneumococcal polysaccharide vaccine to:

a. All children aged <2 years

b. Children aged between 24 to 59 months who are at increased risk for pneumococcal disease (e.g., children with sickle-cell disease or other hemoglobinopathies or children who are functionally or anatomically asplenic); children with HIV infection; children who have chronic disease (chronic cardiac or pulmonary disease, diabetes mellitus, CSF leak); and children with immunocompromising conditions (malignancies, chronic renal failure, nephrotic syndrome, receipt of immunosuppressive chemotherapy, long-term corticosteroids, receipt of solid-organ transplants)

c. Consider administering the vaccine to children aged between 24 to 59 months, with priority to children aged 24 to 35 months, children who are American Indians/Alaska Natives or black, and children who attend group child care centers (IB)

- In nursing homes and other long-term-care facilities, establish a standing order program for the administration of pneumococcal vaccine to patients at high risk for acquiring pneumococcal pneumonia. (IA)

Institute for Healthcare Improvement (IHI) Bundles

The Institute for Healthcare Improvement (IHI) 100,000 Lives Campaign is a national effort to encourage U.S. hospitals to implement changes proven to improve care and save lives. IHI developed the Central Line Bundle, Ventilator Bundle, and Sepsis Bundles to prevent infection and avoidable deaths. A *"bundle"* is a group of evidence-based interventions based on best practice guidelines which, when implemented together, result in better outcomes than when implemented individually.[23]

- Central Line Bundle: Implement for patients undergoing insertion of central venous catheters

- Ventilator Bundle: Implement for patients on ventilator support

- Sepsis Bundles:
    1. Sepsis Resuscitation Bundle: Complete implementation within 6 hours after developing sepsis
    2. Sepsis Management Bundle: Complete implementation within 24 hours after developing sepsis

There are five key measures to fight central catheter-associated bloodstream infection (CA-BSI).[23,36]

Key Components of the Central Line Bundle	
CVC Bundle	**Explanations**
Hand hygiene	Two ways to clean hands before and after insertion: 1. Wash with antibacterial soap and water with adequate rinsing, or 2. Use waterless, alcohol-based hand sanitizer *Wearing sterile gloves cannot replace hand hygiene.*
Maximal barrier precautions upon insertion	The operator inserting the CVC should wear a cap, surgical mask, sterile gown, and sterile gloves. • All hair should be tucked under the cap. • The mouth and nose should be covered tightly by the mask. • The patient should be covered from head to toe with a sterile drape.
Chlorhexidine skin antisepsis (except neonates)	Evidence suggests that antiseptic 2% chlorhexidine gluconate in 70% isopropyl alcohol provides better antisepsis than iodine.
Optimal catheter site selection, with subclavian vein as the preferred site for non-tunneled catheters	Subclavian venous access has a lower rate of CA-BSI than do internal jugular and femoral vein access.
Daily review of line necessity, with prompt removal of unnecessary lines	Conduct a daily review of CVC necessity, and remove unnecessary CVCs promptly.

There are four key measures to fight ventilator-associated pneumonia (VAP).[35]

Key Components of the Ventilator Bundle	
VAP Bundle	**Explanations**
Elevation of the head of the bed	The recommended elevation is 30 to 45 degrees to prevent aspiration.
Daily "sedation vacations" and assessment of readiness to extubate	Include a sedation-vacation strategy in your overall weaning protocol to wean patients from the ventilator.
Peptic ulcer disease prophylaxis	Decreasing the acidity of gastric contents may protect against pulmonary inflammatory response to aspiration of gastrointestinal contents.
Deep venous thrombosis prophylaxis	To prevent pulmonary embolism (PE). *A patient with PE is at high risk to be intubated and placed on a ventilator.*

There are five key concepts of the Sepsis Resuscitation Bundle.[38]

Sepsis Resuscitation Bundle

1. Serum lactate measured
2. Blood cultures obtained prior to antibiotic administration
3. Broad-spectrum antibiotics administered within 3 hours of the time of presentation for ED admissions and within 1 hour for non-ED ICU admissions
4. In the event of hypotension and/or lactate > 4 mmol/L (36 mg/dL):

   a. Deliver an initial minimum of 20 mL/kg of crystalloid (or colloid equivalent)

   b. Apply vasopressors for hypotension not responding to initial fluid resuscitation in order to maintain mean arterial pressure (MAP) > 65 mm Hg

5. In the event of persistent hypotension despite fluid resuscitation (septic shock) and/or lactate > 4 mmol/L (36 mg/dL):

   a. Achieve central venous pressure (CVP) of > 8 mm Hg

   b. Achieve central venous oxygen saturation (ScvO2) of > 70%

There are four key concepts of the Sepsis Management Bundle.

Sepsis Management Bundle

1. Low-dose steroids administered for septic shock in accordance with a standardized ICU policy
2. Drotrecogin alfa (activated) administered in accordance with a standardized ICU policy
3. Glucose control maintained > lower limit of normal, but < 150 mg/dL (8.3 mmol/L)
4. Inspiratory plateau pressures maintained < 30 cm H_2O for mechanically ventilated patients

Figure References

6-1. Thibodeau GA. Anatomy & Physiology. 6th ed. St Louis: Mosby; 2006.

6-2. Courtesy of the Center for Disease Control and Prevention.

6-3. Rothrock JC. Alexander's Care of the Patient in Surgery. 13th ed. St Louis: Mosby; 2006.

6-4. Forbes CD, Jackson WF. Color Atlas and Text of Clinical Medicine. 3rd ed. St Louis: Mosby; 2003.

6-5. Potter PA. Basic Nursing: Essentials for Practice. 6th ed. St Louis: Mosby; 2006.

6-6. Harkreader H. Fundamentals of Nursing: Caring and Clinical Judgment. 3rd ed. Philadelphia: Saunders; 2007.

6-7. Rothrock JC. Alexander's Care of the Patient in Surgery. 13th ed. St Louis: Mosby; 2006.

6-8. Des Jardins T. Clinical Manifestations and Assessment of Respiratory Disease. 5th ed. St Louis: Mosby; 2005.

STERILIZATION AND DISINFECTION

Sterilizing/Disinfecting Items

1. Organic residues (e.g., blood, sputum, tissue) attached to instruments must be completely removed, and all items must be scrupulously cleaned with water and detergent or enzymatic cleaner to reduce bio-burden before sterilization/disinfection processing.

2. Items should not be used if their sterility is questionable (e.g., package damaged, torn, or wet).

3. A chemical indicator, which shows a package has been through a sterilization cycle, must be visible on the outside of each package sterilized.

4. The level of disinfection or sterilization required depends on the use of the items or instruments. Objects are categorized as critical items, semicritical items, and noncritical items[40,41] based on the risk of infection or disease transmission associated with the use of the items.

5. Sterilization/disinfection of items is a complicated procedure requiring professional training to perform appropriately so that patient safety is ensured.

Critical Items

Critical items are those items that enter normally sterile tissue or the vascular system.

Examples

- Surgical instruments

- Cardiac and urinary catheters

- Implants

- Ultrasound probes used in sterile body cavities

- Laparoscopes

- Arthroscopes

Sterilization/Disinfection

- Items require sterilization

- Items should be purchased sterile

- Items should be sterilized by steam sterilization

- If item is sensitive to heat, it should be sterilized with ethylene oxide (ETO), hydrogen peroxide gas plasma, or liquid chemical sterilants

Semicritical Items

Semicritical items are those items that directly contact mucous membranes or non-intact skin.

Examples

- Laryngoscope blades

- Endotracheal tubes

- GI endoscopes

- Anesthesia breathing circuits

- Respiratory therapy equipment

Sterilization/Disinfection

- Items should be free from vegetative microorganisms and have only small numbers of bacterial spores.

- Items require high-level disinfection with chemicals such as glutaraldehyde,

hydrogen peroxide, orthophthaladehyde
(OPA), or peracetic acid with hydrogen peroxide and chlorine.

Noncritical Items

Noncritical items are those items that contact
intact skin but not mucous membranes.

Examples

- Bedpans

- Blood pressure cuffs

- Crutches

- Bedrails

Sterilization/Disinfection

- Items may cause indirect transmission by
  contaminating HCWs' hands and medical
  equipment used by other patients

- Require low-level disinfection using U.S.
  Food and Drug Administration (FDA) regis-
  tered hospital disinfectant to kill vegetative
  bacteria, fungi, and lipid viruses on the
  items

There are five steps involving endoscope disinfection or sterilization with a liquid chemical sterilant or high-level disinfectant.[40,41]

Steps	Explanations
Clean	Physically clean lumen, channels, internal and external surfaces by brushing, flushing, rinsing with water and detergent
Disinfect	1. Immerse endoscope in high-level disinfectant or chemical sterilant; perfuse to eliminate air pockets and ensure internal lumens contact the germicide 2. Expose for period recommended by manufacturer's instructions for specific product
Rinse	Rinse endoscope and each lumen/channel with sterile water, filtered water, or tap water
Dry	Rinse endoscope and each lumen/channel with alcohol, and dry with forced air before storage
Store	Hang vertically to promote drying; store endoscope in a closet to prevent recontamination

Flash Sterilization

- *Flash sterilization* is defined as sterilization of an unwrapped object at 132°C (270°F) for 3 minutes at 27 to 28 lbs pressure in a gravity displacement steam sterilizer.[40, 41]

- Flash sterilization should be limited to emergency situations—for example, to process a dropped surgical instrument when the instrument must be used immediately. The use of flash sterilization must be fully documented.[40]

- Flash sterilization is not recommended for implants because spore tests cannot be used reliably and because safety is lower, increasing the potential for severe infection.[40,41]

- Never use flash sterilization for convenience or time savings or as an alternative to purchasing additional instruments.[39]

- Flash sterilization cannot be used for reprocessing medical items contaminated with Creutzfeldt-Jakob disease (CJD) patients' high-risk tissues (e.g., spinal cord/CSF, brain tissue, or eye tissue). Prion-contaminated items are almost impossible to disinfect or clean and should be discarded.[40,41] Use disposable instruments whenever possible.

Methods for Sterilization and Disinfection of Medical Items and Environmental Surfaces[40]

Methods	Microbial Inactivation	Medical Application
Sterilization	Destroys all microorganisms and bacterial spores	Critical items
High-level disinfection	Destroys all organisms other than small numbers of bacterial spores	Semicritical items
Low-level disinfection	Destroys vegetative bacteria, fungi, and viruses but not mycobacteria or spores	Noncritical items

Environmental Cleaning in Surgical Practice Settings

- If medical equipment or surfaces of the surgical procedure room are heavily soiled with blood, feces, pus, body fluid, sputum, and so on, precleaning to remove contaminants may be required prior to routine cleaning.

- Operating rooms should be cleaned and surfaces should be decontaminated after each surgical procedure.

- Quaternary ammonium compounds are widely used in environmental sanitation of noncritical surfaces (e.g., floors, furniture, and walls).[41]

- After the last surgical procedure of the day or night, wet vacuum or mop operating room floors with a single-use mop and an EPA-registered hospital disinfectant.

- Management of CJD patients in OR:
  1. To eliminate environmental contamination, noncritical environmental surfaces (e.g., operating room tables) should be covered with plastic-backed paper before performing procedures (e.g., brain biopsies) on CJD patients that expose high-risk tissues.
  2. Prion-contaminated paper/waste should be handled carefully and discarded properly.[40]
  3. Use disposable items as much as possible in the procedure.
  4. Incinerate medical items or waste contaminated with high-risk tissue from brain autopsy procedures of diagnosed or suspected CJD patients.

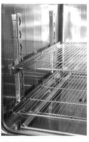
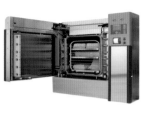

A, Adjustable racks are designed to permit maximum loading efficiency. *B,* Instrument baskets or trays should have either wire-meshed bottoms or a sufficient number of perforations in the sheet metal to allow for air removal and drainage of condensate during the sterilization cycle.

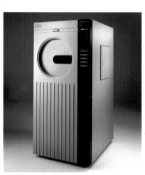

Gas plasma sterilizer.

Figure References

7-1. Rothrock JC. Alexander's Care of the Patient in Surgery. 13th ed. St Louis: Mosby; 2006.

7-2. Rothrock JC. Alexander's Care of the Patient in Surgery. 13th ed. St Louis: Mosby; 2006.

EMPLOYEE HEALTH

Protecting Staff

- Immunization programs protect HCWs from vaccine-preventable illnesses. All HCWs should be immune to measles, mumps, rubella, varicella, and hepatitis B. HCWs should receive influenza vaccine yearly.

- HCWs who are pregnant, immunocompromised, or have certain underlying chronic preexisting illnesses can be given special consideration in immunizations.

The following vaccines are highly recommended for HCWs.[42,43]

Measles Live-Virus Vaccine

Dose:

- First dose, SC

- Second dose at least 1 month later

Indications:

- HCWs born before 1957 who have no evidence of immunity

- HCWs born in or after 1957 with no documentation of:
    1. receipt of two doses of measles vaccine
    2. physician-diagnosed measles
    3. laboratory-confirmed measles immunity

Contraindications:

- Pregnancy

- Immunocompromised status (e.g., AIDS, HIV infected, leukemia, lymphoma, immunosuppression therapy)

- History of anaphylactic reactions after gelatin ingestion

- Hypersensitivity to neomycin or eggs

- Receipt of immunoglobulin

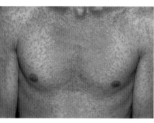

8-1

Measles causes a classic maculopapular or morbilliform eruption.

Mumps Live-Virus Vaccine

Dose:

- One dose, SC

- No booster needed

Indications:

- HCWs with no documentation of:
    1. receipt of mumps live-virus vaccine
    2. laboratory-confirmed mumps immunity;

- HCWs born before 1957 can be considered immune

Contraindications:

- Pregnancy

- Immunocompromised status (e.g., AIDS, HIV infected, leukemia, lymphoma, immunosuppression therapy)

- History of anaphylactic reactions after receipt of neomycin or gelatin ingestion

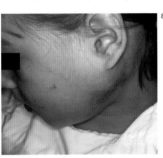
8-2

Endemic parotitis (mumps). Child with painful parotid swelling.

Rubella Live-Virus Vaccine

Dose:

- One dose, SC

- No booster needed

Indications:

- Both male and female HCWs with no documentation of:
    1. receipt of rubella live-virus vaccine
    2. laboratory-confirmed rubella immunity;

- HCWs born before 1957 can be considered immune

Contraindications:

- Pregnancy

- Immunocompromised status (e.g., AIDS, HIV infected, leukemia, lymphoma, immunosuppression therapy)

- History of anaphylactic reactions after receipt of neomycin

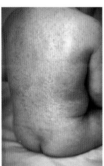
8-3

Rubella rash on a child's back. The distribution is similar to that of measles, but the lesions are less intensely red.

Varicella

Dose:

- First dose, SC

- Second dose 4 to 8 weeks later if ≥13 years old

Indications:

- HCWs with no reliable history of varicella or laboratory-confirmed varicella immunity

Contraindications:

- Pregnancy
- Immunocompromised status (e.g., AIDS, HIV infected, leukemia, lymphoma, immunosuppression therapy)
- History of anaphylactic reactions after gelatin ingestion
- Hypersensitivity to neomycin
- Usage of salicylates should be avoided for 6 weeks after vaccination.

Hepatitis B

Dose:

- First dose, IM (deltoid muscle)
- Second dose 1 month later
- Third dose 5 months after second dose
- No booster needed

Indications:

- HCWs at risk of exposure to blood and body fluids

Contraindications:

- Hypersensitivity to common baker's yeast

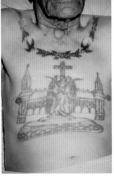

8-4

This patient developed acute hepatitis B after being tattooed in the Far East, and he subsequently became a long-term carrier of the hepatitis B virus.

Influenza

Dose:

- Single dose; IM yearly

Indications:

- HCWs who provide care to high-risk patients or work in chronic-care facilities

- Personnel with high-risk medical conditions and/or age ≥65

Contraindications:

- Anaphylactic hypersensitivity to eggs

- No evidence of risk to mother or fetus when pregnant women receive influenza vaccine

Occupational Exposure

- Occupational exposure poses a serious risk to HCWs. Occupational exposure can be prevented through compliance with Standard Precautions, use of appropriate personal protective equipment, and use of devices/needles with safety features.

- Occupational exposure places HCWs at risk of bloodborne pathogen infections (e.g., hepatitis B virus [HBV], hepatitis C virus [HCV], or human immunodeficiency virus [HIV]) through a percutaneous sharp injury or contact with mucous membranes or non-intact skin.

- Wounds should be cleaned with soap and water. Eyes should be flushed with clean water from an eye irrigator. There is no evidence of benefit in applying antiseptic (e.g., iodine, alcohol) or squeezing the puncture site to force bleeding. Mucous membranes should be washed with clean water.[44]

- Occupational exposure also causes transmission of tuberculosis. The Occupational Safety and Health Administration (OSHA) has regulations addressing occupational exposure to tuberculosis. A tuberculosis-screening program should be implemented based on risk assessment of each facility. The purified protein derivative (PPD) tuberculosis skin test (0.1 mL) should be administered, read, interpreted, and tracked by a trained professional.

- If suspected clinical signs and symptoms are presented, HCWs should be empowered to start proper isolation precautions before patient's diagnosis is confirmed to avoid occupational exposure.

- Facilities should have a multifaceted approach to managing postoccupational exposure, including investigation, intervention, and improvement.

Needlestick Safety and Prevention

- The Needlestick Safety and Prevention Act is designed to protect HCWs from occupational exposure to bloodborne pathogens through accidental sharps injuries in healthcare and other occupational settings.[44]

- Healthcare settings should implement engineering controls (e.g., sharps disposal containers, self-sheathing needles, safer medical devices, and needleless systems) to isolate or remove bloodborne pathogen hazards from the workplace. Also, employees with risk of occupational exposure to blood and body fluid must be trained regarding the proper use of all engineering and work practice controls.[44]

- OSHA intends the sharp injury log to be used as a tool to identify high-risk sharp injury locations and provide information important to sharp injury improvement and device evaluation.

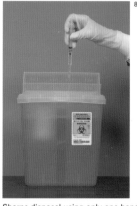
8-5

Sharps disposal using only one hand.

Figure References

8-1. Goldman L, Ausiello DA. Cecil Medicine: Expert Consult. 23rd ed. Philadelphia: Saunders; 2007.

8-2. Sapp JP. Contemporary Oral and Maxillofacial Pathology. 2nd ed. St Louis: Mosby; 2003.

8-3. From Centers for Disease Control and Prevention Image Bank, Figure #712.

8-4. Forbes CD, Jackson WF. Color Atlas and Text of Clinical Medicine. 3rd ed. St Louis: Mosby; 2003.

8-5. Potter PA. Basic Nursing: Essentials for Practice. 6th ed. St Louis: Mosby; 2006.

COMMON HEALTHCARE-ASSOCIATED INFECTIONS

Infections Commonly Found in Healthcare Facilities, *128*

COMMON HEALTHCARE-ASSOCIATED INFECTIONS

Infections Commonly Found in Healthcare Facilities

- The CDC strives to understand the circumstances leading to the occurrence of healthcare-associated infections and develops interventions to fight HAI. The CDC estimates that HAIs account for 1.7 million infections and 99,000 associated deaths each year in American hospitals. The HAI rate has become a measure of patient safety and quality of care. Reducing the rate of HAI is vital to improving quality of care and ensuring patient safety.[46]

- Percentage of HAIs by type in U.S. hospitals (adults and children not in intensive care units, 2007)[45]

Percentage of HAIs that were urinary tract infections	32%
Percentage of HAIs that were surgical-site infections	22%
Percentage of HAIs that were pneumonia (lung infections)	15%
Percentage of HAIs that were bloodstream infections	14%
Percentage of HAIs that were other infections	17%

GLOSSARY

Airborne infection isolation room (AIIR): An AIIR is a single patient-care room used to isolate patients with a suspected or confirmed airborne infectious illness. AIIRs have negative pressure in the room, an air-flow rate of 6 to 12 air changes per hour (ACH), and direct exhaust of air from the room to the exterior of the building or recirculation of air through a HEPA filter before returning to circulation.

Carrier: A host (an individual) who harbors a pathogen but does not display signs and symptoms of illness. The carrier may be in a latent phase of the incubation period as a part of asymptomatic disease or may be in a chronic phase after recovering from an acute stage. A carrier may shed the pathogen into the environment intermittently or continuously, possibly infecting others.

Colonization vs. Infection:

a. Colonization: The presence of a pathogen in an individual (e.g., skin surface, nares, intestines, urinary tract, respiratory tract, or wound) without causing signs or symptoms of infection in the individual. Colonization of a carrier may be a potential source of transmission.

b. Infection: The successful transmission of a pathogen to the individual, with subsequent colonization, multiplication, and invasion. The infected host displays signs and symptoms of infection and can shed microorganisms to the environment and infect others.

Decolonization: Elimination of MDRO (e.g., MRSA) carrier state through use of infection control measures and/or antibiotics. This decreases the risk of transmission to high-risk individuals (immunocompromised or otherwise highly susceptible persons) and to others.

Decontaminate hands: To reduce bacterial count on hands by performing hand hygiene with alcohol-based hand rubs or washing hands with antimicrobial or non-antimicrobial soap and water.

Eukaryote: A single-cell or multicellular organism composed of complex cells having a membrane-bound nucleus and organelles. Includes fungi, protozoa, algae, and animal.

Healthcare-associated infection (HAI): Healthcare-associated infections are infections that patients acquire while receiving treatment for other conditions within a healthcare setting.

Isolation: Physical separation of an infected or colonized host—including the infected/colonized host's contaminated waste and environmental material—from others to prevent transmission.

Incubation: The duration between exposure to a pathogen and the first appearance of evidence (signs and symptoms) of disease in a susceptible host.

Morbidity rate: The ratio of the number of patients infected to the number of persons at risk in the population during a defined period.

Mortality rate: The ratio of those infected who have died in a given period to the number of individuals in the defined population.

Personal protective equipment (PPE): In healthcare settings, PPE consists of a variety of barriers used alone or in combination to protect HCWs. PPE includes face shields, goggles, gloves, gowns, masks, and respirators. PPE is designed to protect employees from serious workplace injuries and illnesses resulting from contact with biological, chemical, radiological, physical, electrical, mechanical, or other workplace hazards.

Prion: Neither a bacterium nor a virus. It is a mis-folded protein particle and is thought to be an infectious agent. The mis-folded prion protein has been implicated in a number of diseases in a variety of mammals, including bovine spongiform encephalopathy (BSE, also known as "mad cow disease") in cattle and Creutzfeldt-Jakob Disease (CJD) in humans. All prion diseases affect the structure of the brain or other neural tissue. Prion diseases cause deterioration of mental function, dementia, muscle twitching (myoclonus), and staggering when walking and lead to death.

Prokaryote: Single-cell organism that does not contain a membrane-bound nucleus nor any other membrane-bound organelles. Bacteria are one of two domains of prokaryotes.

Risk factors: Patients' characteristics, behaviors, or experiences that increase the probability of developing a health issue (e.g., infection or illness).

Virulence: The capability of a microorganism (e.g., a bacterium or virus) to infect a host and produce disease. The virulence of a microorganism is a measure of the severity of the disease the microorganism is capable of causing.

NOTES

REFERENCES

1. Siegel JD, Rhinehart E, Jackson M, Chiarello L, & the Healthcare Infection Control Practices Advisory Committee. Centers for Disease Control and Prevention. *Guideline for Isolation Precautions: Preventing Transmission of Infectious Agents in Healthcare Settings, June 2007.* Retrieved August 09, 2008, from http://www.cdc.gov/ncidod/dhqp/pdf/guidelines/Isolation2007.pdf

2. The Joint Commission. *2009 National Patient Safety Goals, Hospital.* Retrieved October 10, 2008, from http://www.jointcommission.org/PatientSafety/NationalPatientSafetyGoals/

3. Rosenthal MB. Nonpayment for performance? Medicare's new reimbursement rule. *N Engl J Med.* 2007;357(16):1573-1575.

4. Consumers Union. *Alarming MRSA Infection Rates Underscore Need for Public Reporting of Hospital-Acquired Infections.* October 18, 2007. Retrieved August 23, 2008, from http://www.consumersunion.org/pub/core_health_care/005017.html

5. McCaughey B. Hospital infections: preventable and unacceptable. *The Wall Street Journal.* August 14, 2008:A11. Retrieved August 23, 2008, from http://online.wsj.com/article/SB121867229022038907.html

6. Archibald LK, Hierholzer WJ. Principles of infectious diseases epidemiology. In: Mayhall CG. *Hospital Epidemiology and Infection Control.* 3rd ed. Philadelphia: Lippincott Williams & Wilkins; 2004:3-17.

7. Osterholm MT, Hedberg CW. Epidemiologic principles. In: Mandell GL, Bennett JE, Dolin R. *Principles and Practice of Infectious Diseases.* 6th ed. Philadelphia: Churchill Livingstone; 2005:161-172.

8. Gladwin M, Trattler B. *Clinical Microbiology Made Ridiculously Simple.* 4th ed. Miami: MedMaster; 2008.

9. Ritter J. Clinical microbiology. In: *APIC Text of Infection Control and Epidemiology.* 2nd ed. Washington DC: Association for Professionals in Infection Control and Epidemiology; 2005:16-1–16-15.

10. Pagana KD, Pagana TJ. *Mosby's Manual of Diagnostic and Laboratory Tests.* 2nd ed. St Louis: Mosby; 2002.

11. Ritter J. Laboratory diagnostics. In: *APIC Text of Infection Control and Epidemiology.* 2nd ed. Washington DC: Association for Professionals in Infection Control and Epidemiology; 2005:17-1–17-4.

12. Centers for Disease Control and Prevention. *Guideline for Hand Hygiene in Health-Care Settings: Recommendations of the Healthcare Infection Control Practices Advisory Committee and the HICPAC/SHEA/APIC/IDSA Hand Hygiene Task Force.* October 2002. Retrieved August 09, 2008, from http://www.cdc.gov/mmwr/PDF/rr/rr5116.pdf

13. World Alliance for Patient Safety. *WHO Guidelines on Hand Hygiene in Health Care: A Summary.* 2005. Retrieved August 09, 2008, from http://www.who.int/patientsafety/events/05/HH_en.pdf

14. The Joint Commission. *FAQs for The Joint Commission's 2007 National Patient Safety Goals.* Retrieved August 09, 2008, from http://www.joint-commission.org/NR/rdonlyres/DBE1118A-8AC1-470E-8089-B40076999655/0/07_NPSG_FAQs_7.pdf

15. Centers for Disease Control and Prevention. *Guideline for Isolation Precautions: Preventing Transmission of Infectious Agents in Healthcare Settings 2007.* Retrieved October 10, 2008, from http://www.cdc.gov/ncidod/dhqp/pdf/guidelines/Isolation2007.pdf

16. Centers for Disease Control and Prevention. *Sequence for Donning and Removing Personal Protective Equipment (PPE)*. Retrieved October 10, 2008, from http://www.cdc.gov/ncidod/sars/pdf/ppeposter148.pdf

17. Jensen PA, Lambert LA, Iademarco MF, Centers for Disease Control and Prevention. *Guidelines for Preventing the Transmission of Mycobacterium tuberculosis in Health-Care Settings, 2005*. Retrieved August 23, 2008, from http://www.cdc.gov/mmwr/PDF/rr/rr5417.pdf

18. Siegel JD, Rhinehart E, Jackson M, Chiarello L, Centers for Disease Control and Prevention (CDC). *Management of Multidrug-Resistant Organisms in Healthcare Settings, 2006*. Retrieved August 12, 2008, from http://www.cdc.gov/ncidod/dhqp/pdf/ar/mdroguideline2006.pdf

19. Strausbaugh LJ, Crossley KB, Nurse BA, Thrupp LD, SHEA Long-Term-Care Committee. Antimicrobial resistance in long-term-care facilities. *Infect Control and Hosp Epidemiol*. 1996;17:129-140.

20. Rupp ME. Control of gram-positive multidrug-resistant pathogens. In: Lautenbach E, Woeltje K, eds. *Practical Handbook for Healthcare Epidemiologists*. 2nd ed. Thorofare, NJ: Slack Incorporated; 2004:180-187.

21. Riley MMS. A lurking danger: A "bundle" of safety measures available to fight central line infections. *Nursing Spectrum*. April 7, 2008:22-27. Retrieved August 23, 2008, from http://nursingspectrum.netstation.us/ce476.pdf

22. Centers for Disease Control and Prevention. Guidelines for the prevention of intravascular catheter-related infections. *MMWR, Morb Mortal Wkly Rep*. 2002;51(No. RR-10). Retrieved August 12, 2008, from www.cdc.gov/mmwr/preview/mmwrhtml/rr5110a1.htm

23. Institute for Healthcare Improvement (IHI). *Getting Started Kit: Prevent Central Line Infections.* Retrieved August 23, 2008, from http://www.aap.org/visit/IHI.CentralLinesHowtoGuideFINAL52505.pdf

24. Mermel LA. Prevention of intravascular catheter-related infections. *Ann Intern Med.* 2000;132(5):391-402.

25. Pronovost P, Needham D, Berenholtz S et al. An intervention to decrease catheter-related blood-stream infections in the ICU. *N Engl J Med.* 2006;355(26):2725-2732.

26. Nicolle LE. The prevention of hospital-acquired urinary tract infection. *CID.* 2008;46:251-253.

27. Burke JP, Yeo TW. Nosocomial urinary tract infections. In: Mayhall CG. *Hospital Epidemiology and Infection Control.* 3rd ed. Philadelphia: Lippincott; 2004:267-286.

28. Leithauser D. Urinary tract infection. In: *APIC Text of Infection Control and Epidemiology.* 2nd ed. Washington DC: Association for Professionals in Infection Control and Epidemiology; 2005:25-1–25-15.

29. Wong E, Centers for Disease Control and Prevention. *Guideline for Prevention of Catheter-Associated Urinary Tract Infections,* 1981. Retrieved August 22, 2008, from http://www.cdc.gov/ncidod/dhqp/gl_catheter_assoc.html

30. Janelle J, Howard RJ, Fry D. Surgical site infection. In: *APIC Text of Infection Control and Epidemiology.* 2nd ed. Washington DC: Association for Professionals in Infection Control and Epidemiology; 2005:23-1–23-10.

31. Mangram AJ, Horan TC, Pearson ML et al. Guideline for prevention of surgical site infection. *HICPAC/CDC.* 1999;20(4):247-278. Retrieved August 22, 2008, from http://www.cdc.gov/ncidod/dhqp/pdf/guidelines/SSI.pdf

32. Wong ES. Surgical site infections. In: Mayhall CG. *Hospital Epidemiology and Infection Control.* 3rd ed. Philadelphia: Lippincott; 2004:287-310

33. American Thoracic Society and Infectious Disease Society of America. Guidelines for the management of adults with hospital-acquired, ventilator-associated, and healthcare-associated pneumonia. *Am J Respir Crit Care Med.* 2005;171:388-416.

34. Centers for Disease Control and Prevention. Guidelines for preventing health-care-associated pneumonia, 2003. Recommendations of CDC and the Healthcare Infection Control Practices Advisory Committee. *MMWR, Morb Mortal Wkly Rep.* 2004;53(No. RR-3):1-23.

35. Bergmans DC, Bonten MM. Nosocomial pneumonia. In: Mayhall CG. *Hospital Epidemiology and Infection Control.* 3rd ed. Philadelphia: Lippincott; 2004:287-310.

36. Institute for Healthcare Improvement (IHI). *Central Line Bundle.* Retrieved October 10, 2008, from http://www.ihi.org/IHI/Topics/CriticalCare/Intensive Care/Changes/ImplementtheCentralLineBundle.htm

37. Institute for Healthcare Improvement (IHI) *Ventilator Bundle.* Retrieved October 10, 2008, from http://www.ihi.org/IHI/Topics/CriticalCare/Intensiv eCare/Changes/ImplementtheVentilatorBundle.htm

38. Institute for Healthcare Improvement (IHI) *Severe Sepsis Bundles.* Retrieved October 10, 2008, from http://www.ihi.org/IHI/Topics/CriticalCare/Sepsis/

39. Rutala WA, Weber DJ. Disinfection and sterilization: what clinicians need to know. *Clin Infect Dis.* 2004;39:702.

40. Rutala WA, Weber DJ. Cleaning, disinfection, and sterilization in healthcare facilities. In: *APIC Text of Infection Control and Epidemiology.* 2nd ed. Washington DC: Association for Professionals in Infection Control and Epidemiology; 2005:21-1–21-12.

41. Rutala WA, Weber DJ. Selection and use of disinfects in healthcare. In: Mayhall CG. *Hospital Epidemiology and Infection Control.* 3rd ed. Philadelphia: Lippincott; 2004:1474-1522.

42. Sebazco S. Occupational health. In: *APIC Text of Infection Control and Epidemiology.* 2nd ed. Washington DC: Association for Professionals in Infection Control and Epidemiology; 2005:26-1–26-18.

43. Decker MD, Schaffner WA. Vaccination of healthcare workers. In: Mayhall CG. *Hospital Epidemiology and Infection Control.* 3rd ed. Philadelphia: Lippincott; 2004:1382-1399.

44. Beltrami EM, Panlilio AL. Occupational exposure. In: *APIC Text of Infection Control and Epidemiology.* 2nd ed. Washington DC: Association for Professionals in Infection Control and Epidemiology; 2005:27-1–27-10.

45. Centers for Disease Control and Prevention, Division of Healthcare Quality Promotion. *Estimates of Healthcare-Associated Infections, 2007.* Retrieved October 10, 2008, from http://www.cdc.gov/ncidod/dhqp/hai.html

46. Klevens RM, Edwards JR, Richards CL et al. Estimating health-care-associated infections and deaths in U.S. hospitals, 2002. *Public Health Rep.* 2002(120):160-166. Retrieved August 22, 2008, from http://www.cdc.gov/ncidod/dhqp/pdf/hicpac/infections_deaths.pdf

47. Lo E, Nicolle L, Classen D, et al: Strategies to prevent catheter-associated urinary tract infections in acute care hospitals. *Infect Control Hosp Epidemiol,* 2008(29) supp 1: S41-S50.

INDEX